NEXT LEVEL

YOUR GUIDE TO KICKING ASS,
FEELING GREAT, AND
CRUSHING GOALS THROUGH
MENOPAUSE AND BEYOND

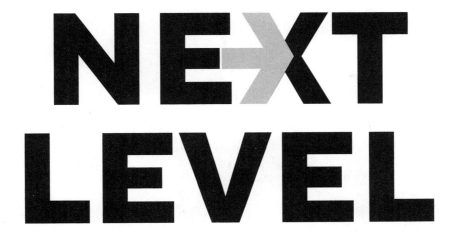

NEXT LEVEL

STACY T. SIMS, PHD, WITH SELENE YEAGER

RODALE

NEW YORK

RODALE and the Plant colophon are registered trademarks of Penguin Random House LLC.

Library of Congress Cataloging-in-Publication Data has been applied for.

ISBN 978-0-593-23315-3
Ebook ISBN 978-0-593-23316-0

Printed in the United States of America

Book design by Jen Valero
Photographs by Linette and Kyle Kielinski
Cover design by Caroline Johnson
Cover photograph by RyanJLane/E+/Getty Images

1st Printing

First Edition

CONTENTS →

FOREWORD

Selene Yeager

For me, the journey to writing this book started with, well, myself.

When I was 43, menopause was the last thing on my mind. I had just come off a jam-packed race season and was gearing up for a big year that would include two massive international bike races, among other huge fitness goals. In addition to all that, I was helping Dr. Stacy Sims write *ROAR: How to Match Your Food and Fitness to Your Unique Female Physiology for Optimum Performance, Great Health, and a Strong, Lean Body for Life*, a science-based training guide for female athletes. I had honestly never felt better or stronger in my life. *ROAR* was published in 2016, when I was 47, and I was still stage racing and feeling pretty good—but I had stopped sleeping like the dead the way I used to. Instead, I'd wake up at 3 a.m. in a pool of sweat with panicky racing thoughts. I chalked it up to work-life stress. My daughter was entering her teen years. Life was getting hectic.

Two years later I looked in the mirror one day and could barely recognize the image staring back. I'd always been a super-muscular woman. Those muscles seemed to have diminished overnight. I'd gained fat in places where I'd never had it. My power was down. I felt sluggish and slow. My periods, which had always been like clockwork, were now all over the map. It was pretty clear at this point what was happening: menopause, or more specifically, perimenopause (but we'll get into those details later).

I'd hit it head on. For any cyclist in the crowd who has ever "endo-ed"—gone sailing ass over teakettle, or "end over end," when the back wheel of your bike flips over the front, sending you headfirst like a spear to the ground—it was a bit like that.

There were the body composition changes and night sweats. I was now having some hot flashes and mood swings as well. Hills that were no big deal in 20 years of cranking up them felt like someone had turned up the volume on gravity. I'd always recovered from hard workouts and races relatively quickly. Now I fell flat when I'd usually be bouncing back.

Even my vagina hurt sometimes. (Seriously, we'll get into that in a bit too.) Once confident and bold, I was feeling the ground shift beneath my feet, like running on an off-camber trail where one slip will send you sliding downhill in a hurry.

Worse, nothing I did seemed to help. I doubled down on going to the gym. I ate less. I did more yoga. Nada. I was still stuck. I'm a realist. I accept that you don't just get fitter and faster till you die. Of course body composition is going to change over the years. But this seemed sudden and intractable.

Damn. Maybe all that shit about being over the hill is true. Maybe I am done. My head swam back into that sea of negativity, through all the stuff I'd heard other women say over the years: "You gain weight no matter what you do. It's impossible to get that muscle back. Nothing helps."

That first book I wrote with Stacy, *ROAR*, had normalized training *with* your hormones instead of just trying to pretend they don't exist. It had included a chapter on menopause, but I needed more information. So I started scouring the internet for resources for active women going through their menopausal years. It was like swimming through a sea of negativity, searching for a flotation device to keep from going under. Everything out there made it sound like the most awful time of life imaginable. The advice that *did* address menopause in a meaningful way wasn't directed at us—active women wanting to stay on top of our game—but mainly at sedentary women. That's because the majority of menopause research is done on sedentary women, who find themselves suddenly at higher risk for heart attacks and other metabolic disease. So the only advice I found was simply "eat right and exercise."

Okay. Got that. And . . . ? There were clearly some gaping holes to fill. So I emailed Stacy. I went on and on, stress-gushing about all the changes I'd been experiencing, seemingly out of the blue. As is her way, she was completely unfazed. She told me about adaptogens with long names that I had to Google a bunch of times before finally getting the spelling right. She told me to dial back all the sets and reps I'd been doing in the gym and to start "lifting heavy sh*t." She informed me that my usual endurance training was fine, but that now, because I was doing more long endurance rides instead of short, hard events, my body was missing the stimulation it needed to prevent the metabolic slippery slope I was on. I needed to reduce the volume and cue up the sprinting, stay out of those gray "kinda hard, kinda not so hard" training zones, and make sure I gave it my all and then went *really* easy to recover.

I took all this advice to heart. I started putting schisandra powder in my coffee, incorporated super-short sprint work into my training, stimulated my muscles with heavy weights, and took other advice you'll find in this book. And it worked. In 2019, at 50 years of age, I won Iron Cross—an arduous mixed-terrain bike race I'd won for the first time 10 years before. I wasn't as fast as I was a decade earlier, but my deeper understanding of how to work with my changing physiology enabled me to feel good and finish strong.

More importantly, I got my mojo back. I felt confident that I could continue challenging myself, growing inside and out, and putting more successful days ahead of me rather than relegating them all to the rearview mirror.

And Stacy and I had the topic for our next book.

INTRODUCTION

For too long, women have been marginalized in the sport science and medical fields. Ever since I was an undergraduate student, I have been asking, "Why?" and trying to find answers to make training and nutrition more successful for my friends and me. As an athlete racing and training at a high level, I also wanted to make sure I was getting the results I wanted from the hard work I was putting in. Once I began asking that one little question, I started hearing responses like, "Why do you want to study women when we don't know enough about men?" So I doubled down and made researching women's specific physiology and fitness and nutrition my life's work. Why? *Because women are not small men!* We deserve research—and answers—all our own.

This was the philosophy behind my first book, *ROAR*, which focused on working with the hormonal fluctuations that occur around the menstrual cycle. Now, in *Next Level*, we'll talk about those topics but really dive deep into what happens as those periods start to come to an end.

This book is for everyone entering, currently in, or already through their menopausal years. As you'll see in a few pages, menopause is just one moment in time: the moment when you've been period-free for a full year. But all the hormonal fluctuations that cause the symptoms we associate with menopause start years—sometimes many years—before that moment. The guidance you need for optimal performance remains pretty much the same from the time you start experiencing symptoms to when you are technically "postmenopausal."

What you're really doing when you act on the advice in this book is picking up the slack and starting to do the work that your fluctuating and dwindling hormones have always done. Simply put, your hormones are messengers that tell your body what it needs to do to stay healthy and strong. They tell your muscles to grow and your bones to form, and they help control your temperature, appetite, and fat storage. As we enter our menopausal years, those hormones start going a little haywire. Some messengers go missing, while others hang around. Some work goes undone, while other functions receive only some of the messages they've come to rely upon. The system is on the fritz. The symptoms that make you feel like you're turning into a furnace in the middle of the night, the MIA mojo, and the body composition shifts are really your hormones sending out a distress call—an SOS signal for you to give them a hand because they simply can't perform their functions the way they used to.

So that's where we come in. There is so much you can do to help those hormones and stimulate positive, powerful metabolic processes in your muscles, bones, and other cells to ease your symptoms. Although throughout this book we talk about the "menopausal" woman, we mean women in peri- through post- menopause.

Next Level is divided into two sections.

"MENOPAUSE EXPLAINED": In part 1, you'll find a deep dive into the underlying causes of menopause: the hormonal changes that are causing all the symptoms you're feeling. We'll also talk about those symptoms—what's "normal," what may require medical intervention, and the impact on your wellness and performance. Once you understand the hormonal players in menopause, you'll be better able to work with them to minimize unwanted symptoms, pump the brakes on many age-related losses, and improve your health, fitness, and performance.

"MENOPAUSE PERFORMANCE": Part 2 is what you *really* came for: what to do about symptoms! This section covers all the ways in which you can work with your changing physiology and maximize your fitness and performance (and ultimately your health and wellness) during menopause. It includes discussions of hormone therapy, nonhormone supplements, strength training, cardio training, pelvic floor and vaginal health, sleep and recovery, motivation and mental health, what to eat, when to eat, how to hydrate, and much more.

We pull it all together with concrete advice for tracking your menopause changes and identifying what's working (and what's not). What we provide here is the framework for your menopause action plan. You'll also find sample exercise routines, fueling strategies, and more. Consider this guidance that you can use for the rest of your life.

And a quick peek behind the scenes: This book is in my voice (Stacy), and I bring the science and research to the table. Selene has shaped the content to make it easily digestible.

CHANGING THE CONVERSATION

We have many goals for this book, but the biggest one is to bring menopause out of the shadows. Too many women feel ashamed to say they are menopausal or to talk openly about this important time of life. Selene and I want *Next Level* to do for menopause what *ROAR* did for menstruation: normalize it!

As Selene shares in the foreword, if you're looking for information from mainstream media outlets about how to maximize your performance during menopause, you'd better pack a snack . . . and some binoculars. You won't find many coaches, trainers, or other experts in the fitness space giving straight-up advice on how to work with your physiology to maximize your fitness during menopause. Few even utter the word at all.

This should come as little surprise when you consider all the negative connotations still carried by "the change of life." There's so much silence because there's still so much stigma surrounding menopause.

Heck, *doctors* barely talk about it. A 2019 study published in the *Mayo Clinic Proceedings* found that of 177 resident physicians in family medicine, internal medicine, and even obstetrics/gynecology who were surveyed, 20 percent received zero lectures on menopause during their training. Fewer than *7 percent* reported feeling prepared to help manage the care of women through their menopausal years. *And that's the modern-day medical field.* Those are physicians, many trained specifically in women's health, we're talking about.

Not long after *ROAR* came off the press, the idea that women are not small men (and therefore shouldn't be eating and training like them) started picking up steam, along with the concept of "period power": the finding that women can actually nail personal records (PRs) and be at the top of their game when they're "on their period." Women came to understand that they feel draggy during certain days of the month, not because their fitness is bad, but because their physiology is shifting in ways that make exercise feel harder. They also learned what to do about it. If you understand your physiology, you can work with it; if you can work with it, you can optimize it.

Just because your periods are slowing down and stopping doesn't mean you have to. We are *way* past the point of valuing women based on the workings of their wombs. Athletically, women in their forties are still in their prime. We see that in inspirational athletes like seven-time world champion Rebecca Rusch, now in her early fifties, who didn't even start her career as a professional bike racer until she was 38; five-time Olympic veteran Dara Torres, who, at 41, was the oldest swimmer to make the team; and Shellie Edington, a 57-year-old CrossFit games athlete who was ranked number one in the world in Masters Women 50 to 54 in 2015, after only picking up the sport when she was 46.

With the right training, nutrition, lifestyle strategies, and the power of the mind (which only gets better with age), women in their fifties and beyond can still chase podiums and elite-level performances. Just ask 56-year-old Laura Van Gilder, one of the winningest riders in American cycling. "I don't look at myself as a fifty-something-year-old athlete," she told *Outside* magazine. "Mentally, at the start line, I'm very much the same as the 17-year-old I'm racing next to, and I want to accomplish the same thing that person does."

We are not going to sugarcoat anything. It's not realistic to say that by following the guidance and advice in this book, you won't face any of the challenges that come with aging. That's nonsense. There are no time machines. But you *will* understand what's going on with your body and you *will* be able to take concrete action to minimize the most disruptive symptoms that come with the hormonal fluctuations of the menopausal years so that you can feel and perform at your best.

Because honestly, I'm not about that whole "60 is the new 40" thing (or whatever the age of the moment is). I believe that you don't need to be younger. We all need to be okay exactly where we are. Forty is 40. Fifty is 50. Sixty is 60. There are a million ways to be 40, 50, and 60 (and 70 and 80!), and we're going to help you be a badass wherever you fall on that spectrum. Sure, at some point, your 5K times are not going to be what they once were. But that doesn't mean you need to put your competitive goals behind you.

From the legendary triathlete Sally Edwards, who at 74 is a CEO, bestselling author, and triathlon hall-of-famer, to the 60-year-old at your local YMCA who regularly laps the high school kids in the pool, women prove every day that our best years can be ahead of us no matter how old we are now.

So to all you forgotten athletes, silent sufferers, and active women daunted by the approaching transition into menopause—enough with trying to stop the clock. That's not the goal of this book. I want to enable you to get through the transition in a positive manner, discovering newfound freedom and power. I want you to be able to say, "Yes, I'm in menopause. Yes, I'm aging. But I understand this transition. I can work with it. I can be strong, and I can do all these new things."

You've accumulated hard-earned wisdom and power over the years. You're higher on the totem pole of life. There are countless opportunities that lie ahead. Let that power and wisdom shine through, uninterrupted by hot flashes, bad sleep, and muscle loss. Menopause doesn't have to be the end of you kicking ass at the gym, on the trail, in the saddle, or wherever you work out. Just bring your health and training to the next level as you reach this next level of life.

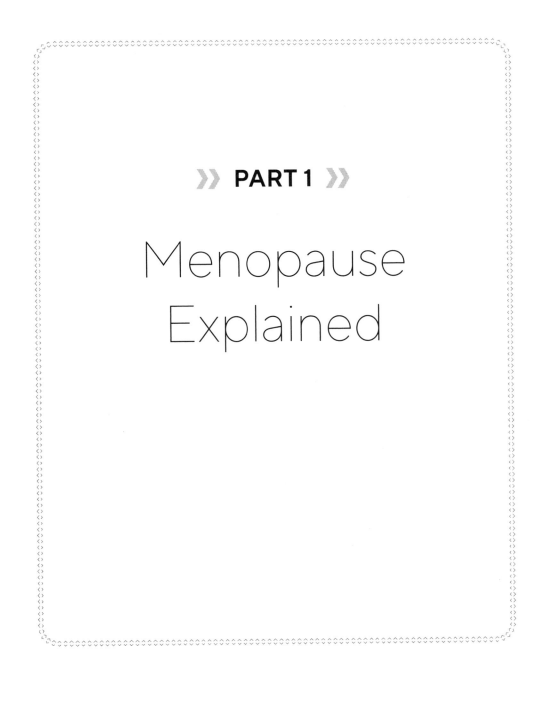

》 PART 1 》

Menopause Explained

1

THE STATS. THE STIGMA.
THE SILENCE.

How we think and talk about menopause matters.

Life expectancy for women is about 81 years, and the average age at which women hit menopause is 51. In other words, nearly 40 percent of your life is likely to happen after menopause. Factor in those five to seven perimenopausal years when your hormones start to go haywire and you could easily be living half, if not more, of your life on some part of your menopause journey.

When you look at it that way, it's all the more upsetting how negative all the messaging around menopause is and has been for centuries. In the time of Hippocrates, menopause was described as "climacteric syndrome," which was understood to be the stage of a woman's life when she had a weakened uterus, was losing power, and was no longer of much use to society.

The Puritan times weren't much better. If you pore through the historical archives on the witch hunts and identify who was killed at the stake, you find that peri- and menopausal women were primary targets. They were "mad with menopause," or they were using herbs and other natural medicines to help treat other women (so they had to be witches), or they were simply "old crones" who needed to be eliminated for the betterment of society.

Menopause finally surfaced as a recognized medical condition in the 1880s, but the terminology didn't improve. It was described as the "death of the womb." The "experts" of the time also believed that when a woman stopped menstruating, she was no longer able to release "toxins," and it was those toxins that would build up and induce symptoms of high heat in the body, profuse sweating, craziness, and "hysteria." The response of the medical community was to call women insane and lock them up.

Things didn't really get much better even in what we would consider modern times. In the early twentieth century, Sigmund Freud and his followers argued that menopause was a neurosis—again implicating menopausal women as insane. The lack of hormones and the aging process were causing women to go crazy. Even into the latter half of the twentieth century, physicians argued that at ages 45 to 50 women were prone to developing hysterical fits. (Don't worry if reading all this is *actually* giving you hysterical fits . . . that's a natural and healthy response!)

Moving into the 1960s, physician Robert Wilson wrote a bestseller called *Feminine Forever*, which described menopause as a disease and "living decay" that should be treated so that women could maintain their youth and sex appeal. That's pretty much what you would expect from a male-centric culture. It was never about us. It was about them.

Fast-forward to today. Though there have been vast improvements in the medical understanding of what menopause is, the messaging in the United States and other Western societies, sadly, has not improved. Menopause today is still viewed as our society's arbitrarily established dividing line between sexual, attractive, and even powerful young women and suddenly old, weak women who can no longer contribute to society.

In fact, even now, women "of a certain age" (a phrase I detest) simply "disappear." We basically stop seeing them represented in popular entertainment. Media outlets like *Vulture* have even made charts showing that as actors like Harrison Ford, Denzel Washington, Johnny Depp, and Tom Cruise get older, the actresses who play opposite them do not—and in fact they are often cast opposite much younger women.

It's no wonder women feel like their lives are over as they age—they're being sent the message that they should just disappear or relegate themselves to the shadows. And when they do finally see some representation, it's often a dated stereotype. Google "menopause" and look at the depictions in the content you find. Compare the depictions of a woman in her sixties with those of men in their sixties. You'll find that there are very different perceptions of what aging is for a man versus what it is for a woman. Rue McClanahan was just 51 years old when she was cast as one of the *Golden Girls*! That's what we're shown on television and in other media: men can still be strong and powerful, maybe even more so as they become "distinguished" with age, while older women are often shown stooped over with a "dowager's hump" rather than depicted as strong, lean, powerful, or attractive.

After menopause, women are usually dismissed. Is it any wonder that women, especially active women who want to be strong and powerful, are so reluctant to talk about menopause?

PERCEPTION MATTERS

How we view aging culturally and societally influences how we view it personally, and those combined views have an impact on how we actually experience menopause, physically as well as psychologically, according to a study published in *Menopause* online, which found that impressions of aging can affect the severity of symptoms.

Lead study author Dr. Mary Jane Minkin, a professor of obstetrics, gynecology, and reproductive health at Yale Medical School, told *Reuters Health*: "In societies where age is more revered and the older woman is the wiser and better woman, menopausal symptoms are significantly less bothersome. Where older is not better, many women equate menopause with old age, and symptoms can be much more devastating."

Taking this idea a few steps further, a 2018 study published in the *Alexandria Journal of Medicine* found a significant and direct relationship between a woman's attitude toward menopause and her body image and risk for depression. Women who had negative attitudes toward menopause were more likely to view themselves negatively and to be depressed. Women with more positive attitudes had better body images and lower levels of depression.

Not surprisingly, poor body image during the menopausal years also ramps up levels of anxiety and depression. A 2020 study of more than 300 women whose average age was 55, published in *BMC Psychiatry*, reported that 55 percent had mild to severe depression and nearly 84 percent had mild to severe anxiety. Poor body image was strongly connected to both.

The catch-22 is that a poor body image can make a person less likely to exercise. After all, if you don't like how you look in your workout clothes, it's only natural to avoid even putting them on, let alone going out in the world in them.

To stay active and feel and perform our best, it's important to break the silence and change the cultural conversation—to feel empowered and more comfortable in the skin we're in and break this negative cycle.

A CHANGE FOR THE BETTER

Menopause is a time to look forward, not back, as the dominant ethos would have us do. Though I'm not opposed to hormone therapy (more on that shortly), I reject the notion that every woman needs hormone "replacement" therapy to stay young. You do not need to recapture something that you have lost. We can use hormones in a positive way to ease the transition, but we should also view the transition itself as an opportunity and a step up—not down—in life.

This is the view in other cultures, especially the Mayan and Japanese cultures. These women go into menopause with a view of it as freeing—they're happy to not have to deal with a period anymore and eager to start a new chapter when they won't have to worry about getting pregnant and being hindered by the responsibilities of a younger, reproductive woman. *The New Republic* did a fascinating feature on the lack of directly translatable words and phrases in the Japanese language for "hot flash," "menopause," and related terms in English. The Japanese experience menopause very differently and—dare I say—positively. Obviously, genetics and lifestyle are factors here. It would be naive to say that it's all in their attitude. But attitude is clearly part of this larger, more positive picture.

Changing the cultural conversation starts with each of us. As part of your quest to be an active, empowered menopausal woman, I challenge you to work as hard on your mindset and point of view as you do on your physical strength and endurance.

THE NEW MENOPAUSE GENERATION

By 2025, more than 1 billion women will be experiencing menopause around the world. Countless millions will be perimenopausal. Countless millions will be post-menopausal.

As an active woman in your menopausal years, you're in some very good company. There are more women in their forties, fifties, sixties, and beyond participating in endurance sports like running, swimming, cycling, and triathlon, competing in power sports like CrossFit, and living active, adventurous lives than at any time in history. According to a report in the *Washington Post* (which cited Running USA, US Masters Swimming, and Ironman), the number of women age 40 and older participating in running races grew by a million between 2010 and 2015; the number of 40-plus women who say they work out with a swim team like Masters swimming increased by more than 25 percent over about the same period; and the number of women 40 and older entering Ironman triathlons skyrocketed from just over 4,000 in 2010 to 10,600 in 2016.

From 2015 to 2018, female (and male) athletes at the CrossFit games have continued to get older. Forty percent of the women's field was 30 or older in 2018, and the discipline increasingly caters to athletes in their forties, fifties, and beyond. (Fun fact: many of the hardest CrossFit Workouts of the Day, or WODs, are named after women as a nod to the hurricane force of these workouts . . . and of women.)

Companies like Machines for Freedom and Nike are now (finally!) showing women with gray hair and more than a few fine lines in their marketing and advertisements. High-profile women like Michelle Obama and Oprah Winfrey are using their platforms with millions (billions?) of followers to pull menopause out of the shadows and into the light. And in a scene that made headlines for its seeming audacity, the actor Kristin Scott Thomas delivered an epic speech on the Emmy Award–winning comedy series *Fleabag*, in which she earnestly and eloquently called menopause "the most wonderful f*cking thing in the world."

So reject negative connotations about menopause. It is something every woman experiences. It's a transition we can lean into and push through as we enter a different phase of life that is full of meaning and wisdom.

Seek out positive images. I know I'm not the only one who is tired of the negative BS surrounding menopause and pushing for change. Besides Oprah and Michelle Obama, other high-profile women like Justine Bateman, Stevie Nicks, Patti LaBelle, Patti Smith, Sigourney Weaver, and Sharon Stone are stepping into the spotlight and celebrating the value of the lessons they've learned with a few decades of life under their belts and the strength that comes with embracing age. Fill your social media feeds with positive menopause images and share your own strong menopausal images. The more we are all seen and heard, the quicker the cultural tide will shift.

Speaking of being heard, use your language and self-talk carefully. The transition through menopause can be hard. Nobody denies that. But if we constantly paint it as a dreadful thing to suffer through, we make it more difficult for ourselves and those following in our footsteps to navigate. If you're constantly looking back and reminding yourself of all the things you used to do, you can't look forward to all the things you still can and will do. Accept the challenge of thriving through menopause just as you would the challenge of running a marathon, completing a triathlon, trying an obstacle course race, or nailing a challenging CrossFit workout. Gather the information you need to succeed, put your best practices into place, follow a program, track your progress, learn from your missteps, and keep showing up for yourself. You got this.

2

THE SCIENCE OF THE MENOPAUSE TRANSITION

Menopause is just one point in time.
The physiology behind it can last decades.

There's a scene in Stephen King's classic horror movie *Carrie* where the protagonist gets her period and thinks she's dying because no one ever told her what those puberty hormones were doing to her body.

Well, the menopause transition can be kind of like that for women who don't get much information from their doctors. You can wake up in the middle of the night with anxious, racing thoughts and heart palpitations, your body dripping with sweat, and think you're dying when what's really happening is perimenopause.

These symptoms can take younger women by surprise, because we think of the transition through menopause as happening in our early fifties—51 or 52 is the national average in the United States—but again, menopause is just one point in time: the point when you haven't had a period for 12 months. Your ovaries start the aging process that leads to that point years, maybe even a decade, before you officially hit menopause. And about 5 percent of women experience early menopause between the ages of 40 and 45, so they can be experiencing symptoms as early in life as their late thirties.

The good news is that, as an active woman, you'll weather the transition better than more sedentary women and may suffer less with insomnia, depression, and other disruptive symptoms. The less great news is that nobody skates through menopause without at least some symptoms that can impede exercise performance and quality of life. To understand what to do about them, it helps to have a full understanding of what's going on.

PERIMENOPAUSE: HORMONAL SOS

Perimenopause is the menopause transition during which you go from your regular cycle of 25 to 40 days, lasting three to seven days, to a very inconsistent cycle. You may miss periods or have heavy, prolonged periods that seem to go on forever. Perimenopause can start as early as 36 but usually begins around age 45.

Why does this happen to your menstrual cycle? Because the sex hormones that have orchestrated the rhythms of your cycle since you hit puberty are now in flux. The primary hormones driving these changes are estrogen and progesterone. During your premenopausal years, your ovaries secrete estrogen to thicken the lining of the uterus as an egg matures inside one of them; the hormone reaches its highest level during the second week of your four-week cycle. Your ovaries secrete progesterone after the egg follicle bursts open and ejects the egg during ovulation; that hormone peaks between weeks three and four. Together estrogen and progesterone are the primary drivers for getting your body ready each month to achieve and maintain a pregnancy.

During the years leading up to menopause, the number of eggs in your ovaries declines, so they're not releasing eggs like clockwork every month. Your body is still ramping up estrogen to plump up the uterus lining, but in a month when a mature egg isn't released, there's no progesterone. So you have an imbalance of too much estrogen and too little progesterone. The next month might be normal, only to be followed by another month or two when no egg is released. In general, imbalance can lead to estrogen dominance, which triggers a host of symptoms, including headaches, mood swings, and more. (You'll find a complete breakdown of perimenopause symptoms in the next chapter.)

This will not be the scenario, however, for every woman. Though less common, some women will experience both a low estrogen and low progesterone state. This happens more often in women who have had really light periods or issues with amenorrhea (missing periods), which is common (though never healthy) among female athletes and very active women. This can also happen among women who have a history of producing low progesterone and estrogen levels during their reproductive years.

These hormonal fluctuations can last up to 10 years, but they're generally felt most keenly during the four to five years before your periods stop for good. Now fully in perimenopausal territory, this is the time when you notice that things aren't as they used to be. In your thirties you may have trained hard and responded well, achieving your performance goals, but then by your forties you notice that you have a little bit more difficulty. You may be thinking, *Wait a second. I'm not able to lose body fat and lean up as quickly as I used to.* And then you reach a point, often in your later forties, when it feels like the training and nutrition that always worked so well for you just aren't doing it anymore. This is when you begin to feel those inherent changes that people talk about as "menopause": you start having night sweats, put on belly fat, lose lean mass, and don't feel as strong and capable of hitting the high intensities you used to. The closer you get to the actual cessation of your menstrual cycle, the worse these symptoms become.

All of this is happening because your hormone ratios have changed and your body is responding to that change. Remember, your hormones are messengers that communicate with nearly every cell in your body, telling them what to do. When those signals fizzle out or get unexpectedly weaker or stronger, the result can be metabolic chaos. The symptoms are your signal to step in and provide assistance. Though it is never too late to respond to these signals by stepping in and taking action to mitigate the effects of hormonal fluctuation, taking action during perimenopause can really have a profound effect. Too many women write off what they're experiencing as just getting older. Some of the changes may be age-related, but a lot of them, like pronounced body composition shifts, poor insulin sensitivity, hot flashes, mood swings, disrupted sleep, and poor energy levels, are hormonally driven and can be mitigated. By acting now, you can maintain performance and make progress toward your athletic goals as you go through the transition.

SHOULD I GET TESTED TO SEE IF I'M IN MENOPAUSE?

Some women ask if they should get tested for signs of menopause. Generally speaking, the answer is no. As readers of *ROAR* know, as well as anyone familiar with my work, I absolutely think it's worthwhile to track your menstrual cycles as they relate to how you're feeling and your performance. I also think it's worthwhile to track your cycles and menopausal symptoms (you can find more on how to do that in chapter 19 as a way to get a picture of what is going on). But getting "tested for menopause" is a little more slippery.

The issue is that you could go in for a blood test at 2 p.m. on Monday and find out that your estrogen levels are high and your progesterone levels are low, but two days later you could get the same blood test done and find out that your levels are "normal." That is the nature of perimenopause. Your hormones are up and down and all over the place, so doctors generally manage your care by asking instead about your menstrual cycle and your symptoms.

Now, if you want to get a better picture of where you are in your journey through menopause, you can get a test to measure your blood follicle-stimulating hormones (FSH). FSH helps control the menstrual cycle and stimulates the growth of eggs in your ovaries. Like all your hormones, FSH fluctuates throughout your cycle and your life, especially as you get older and start experiencing non-ovulatory cycles. That said, FSH can be a fairly reliable indicator of menopause. When a woman's FSH level is consistently elevated to 30 milli-international units per liter (mIU/mL) or higher and she hasn't had a period for a year, it's generally accepted that she's reached menopause. The key words here are "consistently elevated," since a single elevated test isn't particularly meaningful.

You can also ask for a test to measure your anti-Müllerian hormone (AMH) levels. In 2018, the Food and Drug Administration (FDA) allowed the marketing of the picoAMH Elisa diagnostic test to aid in the determination of a woman's menopausal status. AMH is a hormone that is produced in the tiny sacs in your ovaries that house and release eggs. The more egg cells you have in your ovaries, the higher your AMH levels. If you have low AMH levels—less than 10 picograms per milliliter (pg/ml)—you're likely to have your final period within the next year. Your doctor can use this test to measure the levels of AMH in your blood but will still ask about your symptoms and use those as a gauge.

A 2020 study of more than 1,500 women, average age 47.5, found that women age 51 and older with low AMH levels had a 79 percent chance of having their final period within the next year. Women with high AMH levels (more than 100 picograms per milliliter) had a 90 to 97 percent chance (depending on their age) of not having their last period in the next year.

If you look at your FSH and/or AMH along with your estrogen and progesterone ratios, it can give you a bigger and better picture of where you are on the menopause spectrum. But none of it is necessary to begin taking action to mitigate the symptoms you're experiencing.

Regardless of whether or not you have these specific tests done, every woman should get a comprehensive panel to assess broader health, including blood sugar levels, cholesterol and triglyceride levels, a C-reactive protein test (CRP) to measure inflammation, and a thyroid panel (this one is particularly useful for menopausal women, since thyroid function can affect hormone levels and the symptoms you experience), as well as an iron panel and vitamin D levels (inadequate vitamin D can promote iron deficiency during perimenopause).

MENOPAUSE: THE DAY YOUR PERIOD ENDS

Once more, menopause is just one specific point in time—the day you realize, if you've been tracking (and you should be tracking), that you've gone a full year without a period. It's also pretty common to think that you've rounded this corner, then wake up one morning and realize you have to reset the timer.

The average age for menopause is 51 or 52, but some women have gone into menopause as young as 40 because of premature ovarian failure or other health issues. On the flip side are women who have what is called late-onset menopause: by 55 to 60, they are just reaching menopause.

If you haven't been tracking your periods, or you think you're in menopause but have the occasional spotting, your doctor can order the picoAMH Elisa diagnostic test (see the box "Should I Get Tested to See If I'm in Menopause?") to determine whether or not you've reached menopause.

Once you determine that you've hit menopause, the rest of your life is called postmenopause. Hormonally speaking, this is your biological state for the rest of your life.

POSTMENOPAUSE: THE REST OF YOUR LIFE

Contrary to popular belief, you don't just completely stop producing estrogen after menopause. As a woman, you make three types of estrogen over the course of your life: estrone, estradiol, and estriol.

Estradiol (E2) is the main female hormone that you make over the course of your reproductive life; this is the form of estrogen that flatlines completely during menopause. The lack of E2 is the main driver for many of the issues, such as the increased risk of heart disease, that women face postmenopause. Your body increases production of estriol (E3) during pregnancy; the rest of the time, when you're not pregnant, you have only barely detectable trace amounts of E3. After menopause, you primarily make estrone (E1), which is a far weaker form of the hormone than E2. At this point, your ovaries are producing very little estrogen; most of the estrogen you are creating is generated from fat tissue in the form of E1.

Why do doctors often recommend that women lose weight as a way to help manage menopause symptoms? Because excess E1 produced by fat tissue can cause some women to experience hot flashes and night sweats for 20 years or more. Research shows that having a greater percentage of body fat increases your chances of having vasomotor symptoms like hot flashes, sweating, and heart palpitations. If you have excess fat, especially visceral fat, losing weight can help. In a study of 17,473 women going through menopause, those who lost 10 pounds or more had fewer—or eliminated—hot flashes and night sweats over the course of a year than those who stayed the same weight.

The next chapter will take a deeper dive into the hormones as they relate to specific symptoms you may be experiencing, and how these hormonal changes affect different aspects of your fitness, performance, and well-being. And of course, we will also discuss what you can do about it, whether you're just entering or already through menopause.

MENOPAUSE ACROSS RACES AND ETHNICITIES

Lots of factors affect the symptoms you experience as you enter your menopausal years, as well as *when* you enter your menopausal years. Everything from your lifestyle (smoking has been linked to an earlier menopause and worse symptoms) to how active you are to your family history plays a role in your experience with this transition. Less talked about is the influence of race and ethnicity, both of which also factor into when you start and how you experience menopause.

More than 3,300 women have participated in the Study of Women's Health Across the Nation (SWAN), which began in 1994 and is one of the largest and most comprehensive studies of menopause in the United States. According to SWAN data published on EndocrineWeb, women of color tend to enter perimenopause and menopause earlier than their Caucasian peers, have longer transition periods, and experience more intense vaginal symptoms and hot flashes.

While the average age for reaching menopause overall is 51, Black and Hispanic women on average reach menopause two years earlier, at 49. So, as a Black or Hispanic woman, you may experience perimenopausal symptoms sooner than you might expect. Black women also take longer to transition to menopause and appear to experience longer periods of irregular bleeding.

When it comes to symptoms, the average duration of menopause-related hot flashes and night sweats is lowest for Japanese American women, at 4.8 years. According to research, Chinese American women can expect symptoms to last 5.4 years. Non-Hispanic white women generally experience symptoms for 6.5 years, while Hispanic women's symptoms linger for 8.9 years, and Black women can expect more than a decade of symptoms. Average weight is a factor here, as leaner

Black women experience symptoms for a shorter duration than Black women who are clinically considered overweight.

Vaginal symptoms also seem to vary across race and ethnicity, with Hispanic women reporting more symptoms like vaginal dryness.

A separate study of more than 1,500 perimenopausal women, average age of 48.5 years, found that Native American women were the most likely (about 67 percent) to report vasomotor symptoms like hot flashes, night sweats, and heart palpitations, followed by Black women at 61.4 percent, white women at 58.3 percent, Hawaiian/Pacific Islander women at 45.5 percent, women of mixed-ethnicity at 42.1 percent, Hispanic women at 41.7 percent, Vietnamese women at 40.0 percent, Filipino women at 38.9 percent, Japanese women at 35.9 percent, East Indian women at 31.3 percent, Chinese women at 29.0 percent, and other Asian women at 25.6 percent.

There are myriad factors in the different experiences of women of different races and ethnicities, including genes, diet, lifestyle, and cultural expectations, as well as the general stress load that women of different races and ethnicities face. Some have suggested that the prevalence of soy in their diet is a big reason that women in Asian countries seem to suffer fewer night sweats and hot flashes. However, research on soy intake and Caucasian women is somewhat mixed. Some studies suggest that white women who eat more soy have *more* menopausal symptoms like hot flashes. But in reality, it's a chicken-or-the-egg situation: soy is not a large part of the Western diet, and when women in the United States have symptoms, they're told to eat more soy. Women who don't have as many symptoms are not often reaching for more soy.

It's also important to recognize that our genetic and ethnic differences permeate every cell of our bodies. Women of European and North American descent don't metabolize the isoflavones in soy the same way that women of Asian descent do. Research shows that while 50 to 60 percent of women in Asian populations have gut bacteria that can metabolize key isoflavones and produce the metabolites that reduce vasomotor symptoms like hot flashes, only 20 to 30 percent of women in Western countries have that type of gut bacteria.

These findings can give you an idea of what your menopause journey might look like. It's also important to understand when you are likely to go into menopause so you can start taking steps to maintain muscle and bone and ease the transition through diet, exercise, and lifestyle behaviors.

MENOPAUSE WITHOUT EXERCISE

If you're reading this book, chances are you exercise regularly and are an active, performance-minded woman. But I think it's worth taking a peek at what menopause looks like in a sedentary woman.

Generally, the biggest concern expressed by all women, exercising or not, is that their body composition starts changing. They start storing fat in their abdominal area (what mainstream media often refer to as a "menopot," a term I do not care for), and they start losing a lot of lean muscle mass. Women become concerned about losing weight, building muscle, and building and preserving bone density.

We know that the biggest body composition changes happen in the three to four years before you officially reach menopause, as the graphs on the next pages show. You can see fat mass going up, starting around five years out. A dramatic uptick in fat mass happens in the three- to four-year period before menopause. Then it tapers and the curve flattens. Although the further changes you see are more age-related than hormonal, that doesn't means you can't do anything about them if you're already postmenopause (we'll get to that later).

The following graphs show changes in body composition in the years surrounding menopause. (The top line is the 95th percentile, the middle line is the mean, and the bottom line shows the 5th percentile).

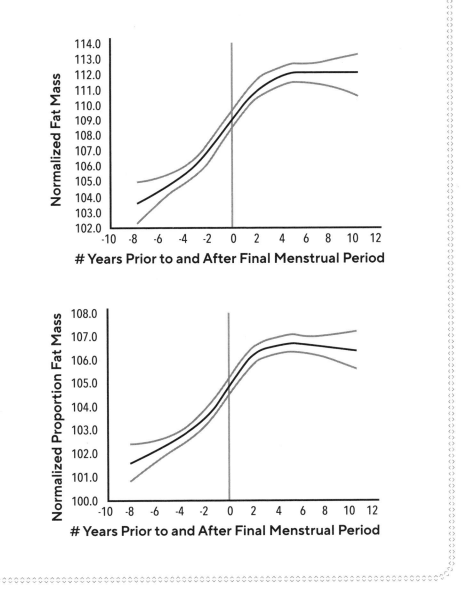

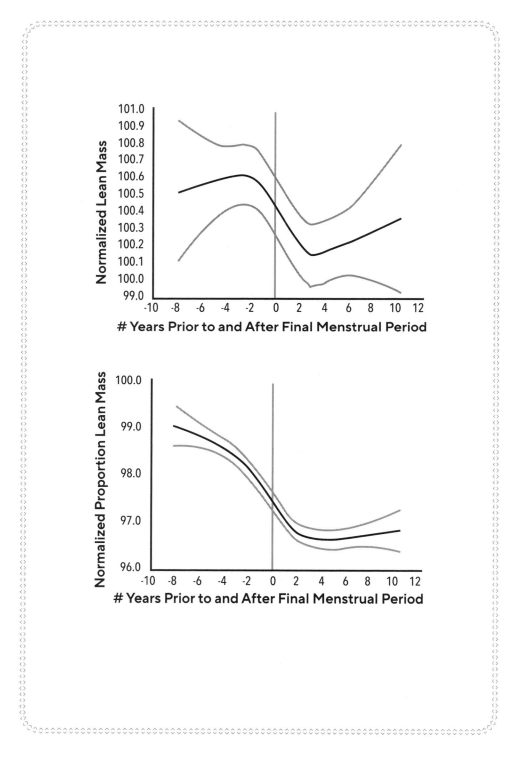

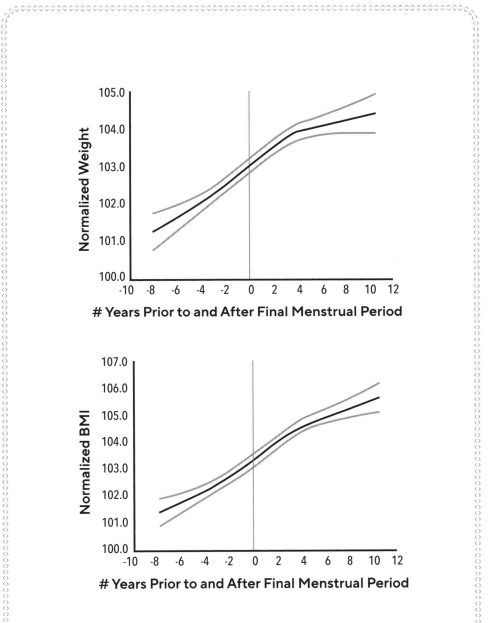

Source: Greendale, G. A., Sternfeld, B., Huang, M. H., Han, W., Karvonen-Gutierrez, C., Ruppert, K., Cauley, J. A., Finkelstein, J. S., Jiang, S.-F., and Karlamangla, A. S. "Changes in Body Composition and Weight During the Menopause Transition." *JCI Insight* (March 7, 2019).

When you look at what's driving these body composition changes, you see decreased insulin sensitivity. So you have higher blood sugar and insulin resistance, which together are a huge trigger for storing fat in the cells and the liver. Add to that elevated cortisol levels from excess estrogen and you have even more factors that will make you gain abdominal fat.

On the flip side, you become less anabolic (less able to make muscle), so your lean muscle is diminishing. And there's a decrease in your bone turnover, so you're losing bone mineral density, which also contributes to the changes in weight.

If you just look at weight increase, it doesn't look as dramatic. It looks like nothing more than a slow creep upward. But when you look at the composition specifically, there's a large increase in fat mass combining with a decrease in lean mass and bone mass.

This graph doesn't factor in exercise. By being active and exercising, you are already reducing some of these changes. But there is definitely more you can do—even if you're postmenopause—to put the brakes on the fat mass gain and muscle loss.

3

HORMONES AND SYMPTOMS EXPLAINED

*How the hormonal havoc
of menopause affects performance.*

Menopause is often referred to as "the change." It's a phrase I've always hated. We are the same person on our Menopause Day as we were the day before. And like "hysteria," it's definitely a term developed by men.

Yes, of course there are facets of our physiology that are changing. We're losing muscle and bone density. We're having night sweats, hot flashes, mood swings, fatigue, achiness, erratic, crime-scene-level periods, and myriad other sometimes bizarre symptoms.

So, yeah. We *know* there's "a change." But because nobody has ever really talked about the root causes of all those changes, women have traditionally been left to deal with them on their own. Gaining fat? Better diet! Fatigue? Fire up the espresso machine! Night sweats? Buy a fan and some special PJs.

And sure, some of those strategies can help. But what we really need is to understand what's going on. Why is all this happening? My life's mission is to understand the underlying why of what is happening in the female body, because it's only when we understand the underpinnings that we can work with our physiology to optimize our wellness and performance. In the case of menopause, that means a deep dive into the hormones running the show.

BEHIND THE SCENES WITH YOUR SEX HORMONES

As you learned in sex ed and biology, you are born with a set number of eggs. Over the course of your lifetime, those eggs mature inside the follicles within the ovaries and are released into the fallopian tube for potential fertilization. If the egg is fertilized, it travels into the uterus to implant so the embryo can grow. If an egg goes unfertilized, the uterus sheds it along with some of the built-up tissue (the endometrium) in what we know as our period and the cycle starts anew.

As discussed in the last chapter, to keep this cycle going, your ovaries pump out estrogen and progesterone to prepare the uterus for potential implantation, and then to shed it should no pregnancy occur. Over time your egg pool dwindles. So, as you enter your menopausal years, your ovaries begin releasing fewer eggs at less regular intervals, and you experience hormone imbalances—your estrogen and progesterone levels rising and falling unevenly as they gradually decline. This change obviously affects the menstrual cycle and is the reason why women in perimenopause can find themselves with terrible PMS, bloating, heavy bleeding, and longer periods.

But the change in your hormone balance affects a whole lot more than just your periods (as if that weren't enough!). We tend to think of our sex hormones as just that—hormones that orchestrate our reproductive lives. But they are *so much more* than that. They help conduct the symphony of our entire mental, physical, and emotional being. The goal of this chapter is to take a deeper dive into these hormones and their role in your health, performance, and well-being. Then, when you get to the next section on menopause performance, you'll better understand the steps and strategies that will allow you to optimize your lean mass, lower your body fat, improve your health and performance, and really raise your quality of life during and after the menopausal transition.

ESTROGEN: THE HEADLINER

Estrogen tends to grab all the media attention. And like any headliner, she can be a bit of a drama queen, especially when left unchecked. That said, estrogen, especially estradiol (E2)—your most potent form of estrogen, as we saw in the previous chapter—plays a key role in a whole host of metabolic functions.

Honestly, it's almost criminal how little women are taught about E2 and its role in their mental and physical health. In the same way that men understand that testosterone is important for their vitality, strength, and overall health, women need to know all the roles that E2 plays in their physiology. That knowledge helps us understand the changes we can make to our nutrition and training plans to pick up the slack when those levels fluctuate and decline, which, as we mentioned in the last chapter, can occur over a period of years, maybe even the better part of a decade.

It's also important to remember that this decline is anything but linear. In fact, it's highly irregular. Two things are happening that impact how you feel and perform: (1) E2 is tapering off, leaving a lot of important work undone, and (2) though your E2 levels are declining, they're not declining at the same rate as progesterone, which as you'll see in a bit works in concert with estrogen. That means you can still have relatively high amounts of E2 (as compared to progesterone; the ratio matters!), even as your total levels decline, and that causes a whole other set of symptoms.

Here's a look at the jobs that E2 does and what happens as it diminishes and gets out of balance with progesterone:

PROMOTING MUSCLE GROWTH AND STRENGTH: This is a biggie. E2 is an anabolic hormone. That means it has a dramatic effect on the structure and function of your muscles. It helps drive the development of lean mass. Without E2, your body isn't as good at building muscle. We'll get into this in detail in chapter 6, but that's why your muscle mass declines so precipitously during this time and why you need to amp up your strength training and lift heavy weights to stimulate and build muscles and make up for the decline in E2.

Likewise, E2 has a direct action on myosin, which is the fibrous protein that acts as the motor behind your muscle contractions. E2 is very important for strong muscle contractions and for generating power and force. When E2 flatlines, the stimulus for those strong contractions is gone. So you need to make up for that loss. Just as heavy resistance training can help offset the losses you experience in muscle building and function, it also can provide the neural stimulation you need to get your muscles' motors revving and contracting strongly again, since you're reproducing the same kind of muscle stimulation in the muscle cells that used to be handled by E2.

SUPPORTING MITOCHONDRIA FUNCTION: Your mitochondria are the power-producers in your cells that turn fuel into energy. All the running and biking and aerobic exercise you do boosts the function of these powerhouses, because the more oxygen you pump into your muscle cells and their mitochondria, the more they adapt to perform faster and better to produce the energy you need for endurance.

There's more to the story where E2 is concerned. Whenever you use oxygen to burn fat and produce energy, you get reactive oxygen species (ROS), or what we commonly call "free radicals": rogue molecules that can damage your healthy cells. Your body, in turn, produces antioxidants that help quench these free radicals so you can recover fitter and stronger. E2 is instrumental in that process, as it helps the mitochondria sweep out those free radicals and makes them stronger. When we lose E2 during menopause, we need to adjust our training and step in with nutritional support to help get the work done that this important sex hormone used to do.

REGULATING INFLAMMATION: Inflammation by itself can be a healthy, natural response to injury or disease. But it needs a dimmer switch so it doesn't go uncontrolled and do more harm than good. That's how estrogen and progesterone work together. Depending on the form of estrogen—estrone (E1) or estradiol (E2)—and the situation, estrogen can be anti-inflammatory or it can promote inflammation. Progesterone is anti-inflammatory. In a perfect world, your hormones work in concert to keep unhealthy inflammation—not the type you get when you twist an ankle but systemic inflammation—balanced and in check. That healthy balance gets out of whack during your menopausal years, when you have more unchecked estrone, which promotes inflammation, circulating through your body.

Those higher, unchecked levels of E1 combine with dwindling E2 and progesterone cause systemic inflammation, which leaves us predisposed to sore joints (sometimes colloquially called menopausal arthritis), impaired gut performance (because inflammation harms your healthy gut microbiome), and fluid retention and puffiness. Inflammation also increases levels of hepcidin, which regulates iron metabolism. When hepcidin is too high, your iron levels can get too low, leaving you with iron deficiency and the fatigue that comes with anemia.

Without our hormonal balance helping us to tamp down inflammation—and all the related symptoms and side effects we experience—we need to take action to quell it ourselves through nutrition, training, and other lifestyle strategies—all of which you'll find in the next section.

MANAGING BLOOD SUGAR: E2 promotes insulin sensitivity, so it helps insulin do its job of shuttling blood sugar into the cells to be stored for energy. It also regulates GLUT4 activity, which pulls glucose into your cells without insulin. As E2 levels diminish, you become more insulin-resistant. It's harder for your body to use starches and blood sugar as effectively as it used to and to get that glucose into your cells. The result is fat storage (hello, sudden weight gain) as your body pulls that blood sugar into fat cells to get it out of circulation.

The good news is that research shows that natural menopause is not a risk factor for diabetes. Even women who are at high risk for diabetes are not more likely to develop it just because of menopause. But managing your blood sugar and energy levels is still essential for your health and performance. Changing your eating and fueling habits (which we'll address in chapters 9, 10, and 11), as well as your training (which we'll address in chapters 5, 6, and 7), can help you balance your blood sugar and energy levels and maintain a healthy weight.

REGULATING APPETITE: E2 regulates your hunger and satiety hormones: ghrelin (the one that ramps up your hunger signals) and leptin (the one that dampens your appetite). E2 itself also acts like leptin in blunting your appetite.

We don't have to tell you what happens when E2 dwindles away to nothing: you lose a major contributor to appetite regulation, which can leave you with more cravings and less satiety. In a 2007 study published in *Nature Medicine Online*, researchers even suggested that "impaired estrogen signaling in the brain may be the cause of metabolic changes during menopause."

MANAGING YOUR MOODS: Remember the discussion in the introductory chapter about menopausal women once being written off (or worse—locked up!) for being "hysterical" or neurotic? Once again, we can point to E2, which increases serotonin, prevents its breakdown, and increases the density and activity of serotonin receptors in the brain. The problem is that your brain gets used to having all that serotonin stimulating all those receptors. As your hormone levels swing and E2 declines, so do your levels of serotonin, leaving those receptors untapped. Your brain is left wanting, which can lead to erratic moods, irritability, restlessness, and anger. Adjusting your diet, exercise, and lifestyle behaviors can help smooth things out.

Estrogen also helps control cortisol, which is commonly known as the stress hormone. We don't have to tell you how you feel when estrogen starts to dwindle and cortisol levels rise: like you're perpetually being chased by some unseen demon even when you're just trying to relax and watch some Netflix.

CONTROLLING BODY TEMPERATURE: Your body likes to maintain a consistent core temperature. E2 helps it do that by managing temperature control mechanisms like blood flow to the skin and sweating. When E2 levels start fluctuating and declining, we lose that consistent control. Your brain overreacts to changes in temperature and senses that it's too hot, even when it's not. So it tells your body to release the excess heat by widening your blood vessels, particularly those near the skin of the head, face, neck, and chest, and release some fluid onto the skin to evaporate and cool you down. The result? The most common menopausal symptoms: hot flashes and sweats.

Hot flashes are always annoying, but when they happen during exercise they can also be a power drain. You need all the blood you can get for your working muscles, and the last thing you want is to feel overheated and to be sweating profusely when it's not warranted. What's more, low estrogen can blunt your normal cooling responses during exercise. Typically, your blood vessels expand as you warm up, sending blood closer to the skin for cooling. With this response dampened, more heat is trapped in your core, so you can feel like you're burning up and need to slow down when you start trying to go hard.

Those changes I talked about regarding serotonin also complicate thermoregulation during menopause. Research shows that the loss of estrogen, the reduced density of serotonin receptors, and decreased serotonin activity contribute to hot flashes and night sweats.

This is where interventions help. We'll cover them in detail later, but I'll mention here that the amino acid beta-alanine helps open your blood vessels before you start exercising, so they're ready to go. Pre-cooling with an iced drink can create a heat sink to take care of that cooking core. Draping an ice-cold bandana over your neck can also help keep you from hot-flashing in the middle of an exercise session.

CONTROLLING BLOOD PRESSURE: E2 helps regulate nitric oxide, a compound in your body that works to expand your blood vessels for better blood flow (which is very important for exercise performance). When we lose E2, our blood vessels become less compliant. They don't constrict or dilate as easily in response to temperature (that is, they don't widen when we're hot and constrict when we're cold), and they don't respond as well when we change our position—going from sitting to standing, for instance.

This effect of loss of E2 can cause your blood pressure to creep up (contributing to your higher risk of heart disease postmenopause). It also can make exercise harder. If your arteries don't dilate as quickly or as fully as you need them to, your heart needs to pump harder to circulate blood, which means you have a higher heart rate even at lower exercise intensities. And of course, high blood pressure can cause serious health problems like heart attack, stroke, and atrial fibrillation (A-fib, or abnormal heart rhythms). Some women also experience dizziness, especially when they stand up too fast. Once again, as women, we need to adjust and work with our changing physiology to mitigate the worst of these side effects and maintain our health and performance.

BUILDING BONE: E2 helps increase calcium absorption, decreases how much calcium you lose in your urine, and regulates key mechanisms involved in maintaining bone turnover and density. So E2 is critical for maintaining bone density and the strength of your bones. That's why it's important to change your training to overcome what you're losing when these estrogen levels flatline.

The typical one-dimensional stress that you put on your bones by running and lifting isn't going to cut it. It's not enough to make up for the loss of E2. You need multidirectional stress on your skeleton in the form of jumping, bounding, and side-to-side impact exercise (see chapter 7 on plyometrics). But don't worry. Anyone can do it, and it only takes a little bit to make a big difference.

KEEPING YOUR VAGINA HAPPY: Estrogen stimulates tissue growth, which helps maintain the thickness of the vaginal lining. It also helps keep the vagina moist. As estrogen declines, the vaginal walls thin and become drier. Sex can start to hurt, obviously, but so can pretty much any other activity. Postmenopausal women may start avoiding cycling, running, and exercise in general (as well as sex) because it hurts. With the right interventions, we can take care of that too!

PROGESTERONE: ESTROGEN'S INVALUABLE SIDEKICK

Progesterone counterbalances estrogen. It pals around with estrogen and tones down the drama. It goes up after ovulation and ebbs and flows with your natural menstrual cycle. During cycles when you don't release an egg, you have higher levels of estrogen, but no progesterone to balance it out. The fewer eggs you release, the lower your progesterone levels become until they hit rock bottom as you enter and go through menopause. Fortunately, your brain also produces some progesterone, so you will have some circulating after your ovaries have called it quits on production.

That's good news, because progesterone not only balances estrogen and helps prepare the body for pregnancy, but it also performs its own important functions throughout the body, including:

INCREASING CONNECTIVE TISSUE STABILITY: Estrogen can loosen your tendons and ligaments, leading to a loss of stability. Progesterone comes in and helps stabilize those connective tissues by increasing the tension on them. When we get into menopause, we lose that counterbalance and our risk goes up for ligament injuries like ACL and MCL tears. Women's shoulders are also very vulnerable to injury.

Many women I work with struggle with stability even at younger, premenopausal ages. They start to do a quarter or half squat, and their knees flare out because the stabilizing muscles and tissues aren't able to keep them in line. Add in the destabilizing effects of changing hormones, and it gets worse. This is why we need to do more stabilizing exercises—to make sure that our supporting muscles stay strong and we can do dynamic, higher-impact exercises to stay strong and build bone. (You'll find all the details on those exercises in chapter 14.)

PROTECTING THE BRAIN: Progesterone is so good for your gray matter that it's sometimes referred to as a "neurosteroid." It produces a calming, anti-anxiety effect in the brain and may enhance memory function. It also increases brain-derived neurotropic factor (BDNF), a protein that has been described in the literature as "fertilizer for the brain."

As progesterone levels decline, we lose some of those important benefits and can have mood swings, memory loss, and the fuzzy-headedness that many menopausal women describe as "brain fog." One study published in the journal *Menopause* found that 44 percent of perimenopausal and 42 percent of postmenopausal women reported being bothered by forgetfulness. The good news is that research suggests that these cognitive bumps in the road are most pronounced during perimenopause and early postmenopause; in many women brain fog dissipates on its own over time (though, again, we have some nutrition and lifestyle advice to help chase it out sooner).

PROVIDING PAIN RELIEF: When progesterone levels are high during our menstrual cycle and in pregnancy, we have a greater pain tolerance. (Makes sense, right?) The sex hormones testosterone (which women have in small amounts) and progesterone (which premenopausal women have in larger amounts) are known to have pain-diminishing properties. Much of this pain relief is the result of progesterone's effects in the brain. High progesterone levels help you feel less emotional about pain—a quality that helps prevent pain from amplifying—and allows you to dissociate yourself from pain intensity and unpleasantness, according to the literature.

It's not a small effect. Researchers studying women with the chronic pain disorder fibromyalgia found that fluctuations in progesterone levels altered their pain levels by as much as 25 percent. That study also found that low progesterone combined with high levels of the stress hormone cortisol (which is commonly high in women during their menopausal years) produced the highest pain levels. Pain levels were at their worst when sex hormones were their lowest across the board.

So if everything seems to hurt more than it used to, the hormonal shift may be to blame. Of course, not every woman experiences this shift. Some women maintain their same pain tolerance because their body has experienced pain enough times through training, maybe childbirth, and life in general that their brains have just come to understand and deal with painful sensations regardless of what progesterone and other hormones are doing.

BUILDING BONE: It's little wonder that menopause is such a precarious time for skeletal health when you consider that both estrogen and progesterone help build and maintain bone density. Like estrogen, progesterone decreases the rate of bone resorption and reduces the loss of calcium in our urine. So when we lose progesterone and E2, we lose powerful stimuli for putting down stronger bones. This is why it's especially important to adjust your exercise, training, stress, and nutritional strategies during this time of life if you want to avoid brittle bones down the road.

HEART RATE VARIABILITY: The last thing I want to get into is the effect of progesterone on our autonomic nervous system and on what we call "cardiac vagal tone." Your vagal tone is a good indicator of how well your body can relax after a stress.

High vagal tone indicates that your resting heart rate is low, and low vagal tone means that your resting heart rate is elevated. One of the most popular measures of cardiac vagal tone is heart rate variability (HRV), which you may see if you have a Whoop Strap, Oura Ring, or other recovery tracking device.

Your HRV is the result of the interplay between the parasympathetic (rest-and-digest) and sympathetic (fight-or-flight) branches of your automatic nervous system. It describes the variability in the time between your heartbeats. When your HRV increases, that means your body is resilient to stress. When it decreases, you have less stress resilience because your lower vagal tone has already put your heart rate under the influence of more sympathetic activity.

This is a complicated metric for women, who during the menopause transition especially have increased anxiety and sympathetic drive. Many women tell me that they use HRV for tracking recovery. But the devices they're using are not based on an algorithm that understands hormone fluctuations, so they can get a false low-recovery score, telling them they are not fully recovered, when they are.

Why? Because progesterone has conflicting effects in the body. It is "calming" in the brain, but has the opposite effect on the vagal nerve and overrides estrogen's effect on increasing vagal tone. In naturally cycling women, when progesterone goes up, estrogen is still there, but progesterone is the dominant hormone. When progesterone drops, estrogen becomes the dominant hormone, which increases vagal tone. In perimenopausal women, the hormone ratios are completely different, and in postmenopausal women, they are flatlined, so the hormonal influences on the vagal nerve are altered.

In plain language, that means you end up with more fight-or-flight activity and less rest-and-digest activity, especially after menopause. To increase your HRV you need to step in and activate those parasympathetic responses with changes to your lifestyle and behavior.

That's important because otherwise we are more predisposed to sympathetic drive and anxiety and less inclined to parasympathetic drive and a lower level of stress, with an overall negative impact on our health and performance.

HORMONES AND YOUR FLUTTERING HEART

Generally speaking, heart palpitations—a feeling of skipped heartbeats, fluttering, or flip-flopping in your chest—are relatively common in women. Along with other arrhythmias and irregular heartbeats, palpitations are particularly common during perimenopause—occurring in about 25 percent of women during the menopausal transition—because all the hormonal fluctuations can overstimulate the heart. It's widely reported that menopause heart palpitations can increase heart rates by up to 16 beats per minute or more.

Palpitations are usually harmless, but you should always get checked out with your doctor anytime you experience heart symptoms like palpitations. The research on menopausal hormone therapy (MHT) and heart palpitations is mixed, so again, have a conversation with your doctor if you are taking MHT or are interested in MHT. Otherwise, general stress-reducing interventions can help, as can reducing caffeine intake and cutting back on alcohol.

MAINTAINING BODY TEMPERATURE: Progesterone increases core body temperature (by about 1.0° Fahrenheit/0.5° Celcius when it's high during the menstrual cycle), while estrogen has a cooling effect. As progesterone decreases, your core body temperature drops to a level more like that of a man's after menopause; some researchers suggest that this change may contribute to midlife weight gain. Also, as your hormones enter a state of erratic fluctuation, your hypothalamus (the thermostat in the brain) gets mixed signals between the environment and your core temperature based on what your hormones are telling it, which can trigger hot flashes, sweating, flushing, and chills.

As you may have noticed, your diet can contribute to these episodes as well. Without progesterone gradually bringing your temperature up and being countered by estrogen on a regular basis, your brain can overreact when you introduce something that heats up your core. That's why spicy food, caffeine, hot beverages, hot baths, sweltering weather, red wine (or for some, any alcohol), dense protein like red meat, and yes, even exercise can trigger hot flashes.

The good news is that there are plenty of strategies for helping the body feel comfortably cool no matter your hormone levels and for reducing the triggers for hot flashes. (You'll find those in chapter 19.)

COOLING INFLAMMATION AND SUPPRESSING IMMUNITY: As mentioned earlier, progesterone generally quells inflammation. It inhibits the inflammatory responses of your innate immune system. Your innate immune system is made of defenses against infection that can be activated immediately once a pathogen attacks. Think about allergies to pollens: the pollen enters the body and *boom*—you've got a runny nose, you're sneezing, and your eyes are itchy. These are symptoms of histamines being released to cause inflammation and draw other immune cells to the fight to get rid of the pollen. This is a good thing. As progesterone increases after ovulation, it suppresses your immune system, so your body doesn't attack an implanted egg as an invader should you get pregnant. It bears repeating that as progesterone levels slide, it's important to find ways to mitigate your unchecked inflammation so that you can protect your iron stores, preserve your joint health, and reduce the risk of the metabolic disorders, like heart disease, that come with systemic inflammation.

BREAKING DOWN MUSCLE TISSUE: Estrogen, as mentioned earlier, is anabolic: it stimulates lean muscle mass development. Progesterone, being the counterbalance, is catabolic. Its goal is to make sure an implanted embryo will survive, so it breaks down carbohydrates to provide energy and breaks down protein into free amino acids, which your body uses as basic building blocks for the uterine lining.

TESTOSTERONE: THE SUPPORTING ACTOR

Women make far less testosterone than men, but it plays an important role. It works in concert with estrogen and progesterone to maintain healthy bones and muscles. It fires up your sex drive and helps protect your brain.

Though your ovaries and adrenal glands continue to produce testosterone even as your other sex hormones decline, building and maintaining muscle is still difficult because of all the other changes that make us less sensitive to the muscle-making stimulus of general exercise and eating protein. Muscle tissue starts to be marbled with fat tissue during this time, which is why women may notice that their muscle tone has changed and their power and ability to recover is lower, even though they are still training the same way. This is another reason we need to change the way we train and fuel to build and maintain muscle and still be able to produce power and recover from hard efforts.

COMMON MENOPAUSE SYMPTOMS

Once you understand the massive role these hormones play in nearly every bodily function, it becomes clear why the menopausal transition can be so disruptive! Not everyone experiences every symptom, but some women's lives are so disrupted they feel like they've been the victims of a hostile hormonal takeover that leaves them trapped inside a body and mind they barely recognize.

Here's a snapshot of the most common menopausal symptoms, what's driving them, and a snapshot of what to do about them (we'll cover training strategies in the performance section):

HOT FLASHES

Probably the most "iconic" symptom of menopause is the hot flash. About 75 to 80 percent of North American women will experience these sudden waves of heat in the face, neck, and torso that can be accompanied by beet-red flushing, copious sweating, and a racing heartbeat. Night sweats are associated with hot flashes that occur at night.

Researchers are still working on understanding all the underlying causes of hot flashes. One known culprit is serotonin. When estrogen drops, so does serotonin. Through a chain of chemical reactions, your brain gets the signal that your core body temperature is too high, so it triggers a hot flash, which sends blood surging to your skin to cool you back down.

That's why antidepressants called selective serotonin reuptake inhibitors (SSRIs), like citalopram, or Celexa, can be very effective against hot flashes, even if you don't have depression. Hormone therapy—low doses of estrogen or estrogen plus progesterone—can also effectively ease hot flashes and night sweats. (We'll get into hormone therapy in more detail in the next section.)

Other drugs that are often prescribed "off label" for hot flashes include certain high blood pressure medications and drugs for sex hormone–related disorders. You can find a breakdown of those in chapter 4.

WEIGHT GAIN

As hard as we work on self-acceptance and body positivity, this is the one that hits many active women the hardest. For our entire lives we've heard about the importance of "diet and exercise" for maintaining our weight. Maybe after years of hard work, we've dialed in an ability to maintain our happiest weight that yields the best performance. But then *wham*, seemingly overnight, we start gaining weight. The average weight gain is about five to eight pounds, though some women gain more. Because estrogen promotes fluid retention (while progesterone decreases it), you can end up feeling puffier too, especially when you're in that perimenopausal phase, when estrogen is high and progesterone is low. All of these changes can leave you feeling weighed down in more ways than one.

Even if we don't gain weight, our body composition changes: we lose muscle and put on fat, and often in places we never had it before. Changes in estrogen and stress hormones send fat to our abdominal area. This is one of the reasons why women's risk for heart disease rises at this time. According to a 2021 study published in *Menopause*, women who put on more abdominal fat during the menopause transition are at greater risk of heart disease (even if they don't gain weight) because of abdominal fat's impact on inflammation and metabolism. The researchers found that for every 20 percent increase in abdominal fat, the carotid artery lining became 2 percent thicker, something the researchers noted could be missed if doctors are only looking at BMI. Carotid artery thickness is an early indicator of heart disease.

The good news is that, as a woman, you also have some protective fat. There's a saying that "thick thighs save lives." Well, there's some truth to that. Past research has found that women with a large hip circumference have a lower risk for heart disease, and a study from 2020 reported that large thigh circumference may be linked to lower blood pressure and a reduced risk for heart disease (and that was in people who were diagnosed as overweight).

In women specifically, large thighs tend to reduce heart disease risk because after the ovaries stop producing estrogen, the main source of estrogen production becomes your fat stores. The problem is that the estrogen produced by fat is estrone, the weaker, less beneficial form, so it doesn't provide the same protection. The estrone produced from the hip and thigh fat stores, however, converts to the more protective estradiol, which is what provides cardiovascular protection for premenopausal women.

Estradiol is so protective that a 2021 study of more than 11,400 men and women published in the *Journal of the American Heart Association* reported that while men and women who have high muscle mass are less likely to die from heart disease, women who have higher levels of body fat, regardless of their muscle mass, seemed to have a greater degree of protection than women with less fat. In fact, women with high body fat and high muscle mass had a 42 percent lower risk of dying from heart disease than women who had low muscle mass and low body fat. The researchers surmised that fat in the hips and thighs may provide enough protection to offset the risks that come with additional belly fat.

This interesting study made a lot of headlines. The researchers didn't look at just visceral abdominal fat—a known risk factor for heart disease—nor did they study only an athletic population. So the main message for both health and performance is to establish a healthy body composition, with an emphasis on putting on and maintaining as much protective and powerful muscle as you can, which will allow you to feel strong and perform well, along with being as healthy as possible, during and past menopause. The next section of this book is devoted to helping you do just that.

HEAVY PERIODS

You would think that as you move closer to the time when your periods are ending for good, those periods would become lighter and less frequent, right? Think again. Many women experience the opposite—heavy periods that leave them searching for enough pads, tampons, or opportunities to empty their cups just to make it through the day.

In a 2014 study of more than 1,300 women between the ages of 42 and 52 titled "Menstruation and the Menopausal Transition," researchers found that it was not uncommon for women to have prolonged bleeding for 10 days or more, spotting for six or more days, and/or heavy bleeding for three or more days during the transitional years. More than one-quarter of women had as many as three episodes of 10-plus days of bleeding over a six-month period, and more than three-quarters recorded three or more days of heavy flow.

Why do periods sometimes get heavier at this time? To borrow an analogy from Dr. Mary Jane Minkin, a menopause specialist and Yale professor, it happens because we have too much fertilizer without enough "trimming." If you think of your uterus as a lawn, the estrogen fertilizes it and promotes tissue growth and thickening of the lining. Progesterone is the lawn mower that thins that lining. When you have anovulatory cycles when progesterone isn't released, you end up with a heavy lawn that hasn't been mowed in a while, and when it finally is, the result is heavy bleeding. Progestin pills can minimize and regulate your bleeding, as can low-dose birth control pills that are mostly progestin (which is very similar to our natural progesterone) with a bit of estrogen. Some women also have success with an intra-uterine device (IUD), which releases small amounts of progestin into the system.

INCONTINENCE

Whether you're out for a run and come back with damp underpants or you are fumbling for your keys and find yourself peeing on the front porch, some form of urinary incontinence happens to the best of us as our hormones decline and take the strength, elasticity, and integrity of our pelvic floor muscles with them. Nearly half of women over 50 say they sometimes leak urine, according to a National Poll on Healthy Aging.

So yes, incontinence is common, but don't confuse common with inevitable—you don't have to just live with it. Performing Kegel exercises (clenching your muscles as though you're "holding it" when you have to pee) several times a day can help. But that's not enough. You also need strong core muscles. Because when your core muscles are weak, your pelvic floor muscles need to pick up the slack and they're not equipped to handle that load—especially if you're running a 10K or jumping rope in CrossFit. Breathing exercises that engage the diaphragm help too. You'll find core strengthening exercises and exercises specifically designed to stop the leaks in chapter 14.

VAGINAL PAIN

As estrogen decreases, our lawn (to use the earlier analogy) becomes a bit less lush, so to speak. Our vaginal walls can become drier, thinner, and irritated, which pretty much makes everything from sexual activity to riding a bike hurt. A Healthy-Women survey of women ages 40 to 84 found that more than half of postmeno-pausal women (56 percent) experienced vaginal dryness and, among those women, 83 percent said that it bothered them.

You really don't need to let it bother you at all, because it is very treatable. Low-dose vaginal estrogen is highly effective at treating dryness. (Remember, estrogen is a vasodilator; when you lose it, you get less blood flow everywhere—including your vaginal tissues.) It's available in various forms, including creams, tablets, and an estrogen-infused ring. Research shows that these products are very effective for improving the health of your vaginal tissues, increasing moisture, improving the vaginal microbiome, and relieving urinary incontinence symptoms. These products do not raise your systemic estrogen levels, so even women who have breast cancer, have had it in the past, or are at high risk for breast cancer can use them.

You also can buy vaginal moisturizers (like Replens and Revaree) that contain a bioadhesive that attaches to the dry cells in your vaginal walls and pulls moisture into them. It can make you feel better instantly and lasts up to three days before you need to reapply.

FATIGUE

Lots of women feel very run-down and tired, especially during perimenopause, when hormonal havoc is messing with their sleep and disrupting their normal energy production. As estrogen drops, cortisol rises, which can be a serious energy drain.

Fortunately, the same exercise, nutrition, and lifestyle steps you'll take to work with your changing physiology and make up for your dwindling hormones (coming up in part 2) should also help boost your energy levels back up to where they belong.

BRAIN FOG

Difficulty concentrating, memory lapses, and general fuzzy-headedness are very common during the transition into menopause because your hormones and neurotransmitters (brain messengers) are in a state of upheaval.

The good news is that brain fog tends to dissipate on its own and cognition stabilizes as your body adjusts to its new state of being. Exercise, sleep, and a nutrient-dense diet also help to clear the cobwebs and improve cognition. We cover these strategies and more in part 2.

ANGER AND AWFUL MOODS

As your hormone levels decline they can drag your mood down with them, leaving you feeling anxious, sad, or angry at levels that may be out of proportion with whatever is happening in your life at the time. About 20 percent of menopausal women also report feeling dyspnea, or labored breathing, which can set up a vicious cycle of anxiety and shortness of breath, according to research.

Stress management is very important, as runaway stress can make mood issues much worse. Yoga, meditation (apps like Headspace can help if you don't know where to start), and breathing exercises can all reel in your stress and anxiety. (Chapter 15 takes a deeper dive into stress management.) Heavy strength training and high-intensity interval training (HIIT) can also do wonders to blow out stress and elevate your mood. Some women find relief with antidepressants (which can also help with other symptoms, like hot flashes).

SLEEP DISRUPTION

Hot flashes, night sweats, and racing thoughts in the middle of the night can all do a real number on your sleep. About half of women transitioning to menopause will have sleep problems. It doesn't help that levels of melatonin, your body's sleep hormone, decrease along with estrogen and progesterone.

Besides taking the usual advice to avoid caffeine past midafternoon, keep your bedroom cool and dark, and avoid alcohol in the evening, you can help your body cool down and get ready for a good night's sleep by drinking a cold glass of tart cherry juice, a melatonin booster, 30 minutes before bed.

Also avoid eating within two hours of bedtime. Making your body work on digestion interferes with the parasympathetic needs of sleep. Have your last meal earlier to give yourself plenty of time to digest so you can get proper rest. (See chapter 13 for a full sleep-promoting plan.)

HEADACHE AND MIGRAINE

Drops in estrogen can trigger migraine headaches through a combination of factors, including changes in blood vessels, blood pressure, and serotonin levels, which is why menopause can actually bring welcome relief for women who have suffered splitting headaches along with their menstrual cycle every month.

But unfortunately, the hormone swings leading up to menopause may make things worse before they get better. A 2016 study published in *Headache: The Journal of Head and Face Pain* looked at headaches among 3,664 women, with an average age of 46. The authors reported that the risk for high-frequency headache, 10 or more days with headache per month, significantly increased in middle-aged women with migraine during perimenopause. Using MHT to stabilize hormone levels can provide relief for some (though not all) women, as can antidepressants.

SO. MANY. SYMPTOMS.

You have hormone receptors on every organ in your body, so when your hormones start swinging and declining, every part of your body is affected. We hear a lot about certain symptoms like hot flashes and body composition changes, and obviously your menstrual cycle becomes more irregular, but there are *many* common symptoms associated with menopause. Here is a fairly comprehensive list of what you may experience during this time of life. We can't promise that we can make every single symptom go away, but we sure can make things a whole lot better!

Hot flashes

Light-headedness

Headaches

Irritability

Depression

Feeling unloved

Anxiety

Mood changes

Sleeplessness

Unusual tiredness or fatigue

Backache

Joint pain

Breast tenderness

Loss of mojo or motivation

Increase in breast size

Muscle pain

New facial hair

Dry skin, itchiness

Crawling feelings on the skin (formication)

Tingling, pins and needle sensations in extremities

Decreased sexual sensation/ trouble with orgasm

Low libido

Dry vagina, thinning vaginal walls

Painful or uncomfortable intercourse

Increased urinary frequency

Urinary incontinence

Increased gas and bloating

Bleeding gums

Brittle nails

Hair thinning or loss

Heart palpitations

Burning tongue

Hearing loss and/or tinnitus

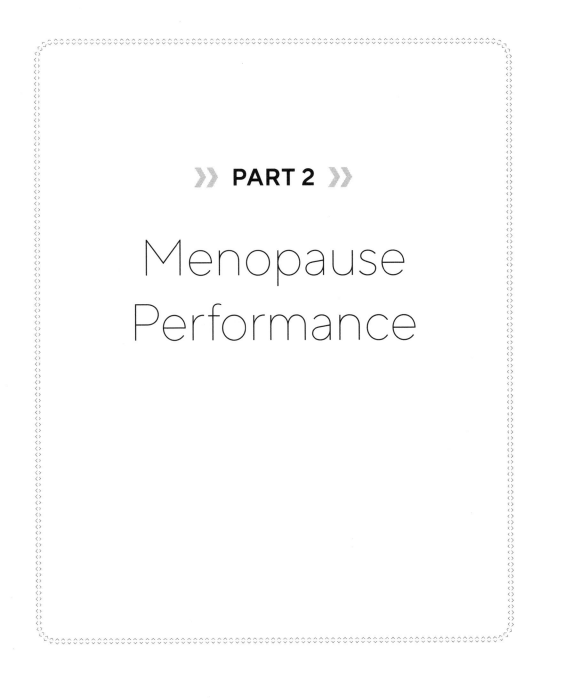

>> **PART 2** >>

Menopause Performance

4

MENOPAUSAL HORMONE THERAPY, ADAPTOGENS, AND OTHER INTERVENTIONS

Some women benefit from additional assistance.

I was going to save this chapter for last but decided instead to address sooner than later what may be the most common question women have at this stage of life. One of the first things most women wonder when they are blindsided by all of these symptoms is whether they should try menopausal hormone therapy (MHT) or other pharmaceutical or nonpharmaceutical treatments to feel and perform better.

The heart and soul of this book is my philosophy that women can (and should) work with their unique physiology to maximize their performance. My ultimate goal is to help you adapt your training, nutrition, recovery, and lifestyle to optimize your performance through menopause, and ideally you could do this without pharmaceutical interventions.

But there is a place for MHT, so it's also important to talk about various therapies that can help your body get through this transitional period. You can be doing everything right and still have full-body achiness that makes it nearly impossible to nail your workouts, or persistent hot flashes and night sweats that disrupt your sleep and your life so much that you can barely think about proper meal preparation.

Even if you are moving through the menopausal transition pretty smoothly, you may benefit from certain adaptogens, which are plants that can increase your body's resistance to stress. That's especially important during perimenopause when cortisol levels naturally rise as the usual hormones that keep them in check are dwindling.

The goal here is to help you understand your options so that you can have informed conversations with your doctor about what interventions (if any) might be right for you. Here's what you need to know.

MENOPAUSAL HORMONE THERAPY

We'll start with menopausal hormone therapy. Take note, I'm not calling it hormone replacement therapy (HRT), because we're not actually trying to replace anything. We are helping our bodies get through this transitional period by supplying low levels of hormones to even things out. We're not actually replacing all the hormones that our bodies were making. MHT is similar to taking an oral contraceptive pill, which is a synthetic hormone that mimics some of the functions that your natural hormones would do.

Before we get too far in, let's take care of the elephant in the room: the perceived health risks associated with MHT. In the early 2000s, the Women's Health Initiative (WHI) from the United States and the Million Women Study from the United Kingdom published some research that scared millions of women away from using hormones during menopause. Twenty years later, many women are still scared, though they really don't need to be. Cautious and smart, yes. Scared, no.

In short, those studies reported that the extended use of MHT might increase the risk of breast cancer, heart disease, and stroke. When this hit the press, everyone freaked out, and many women decided, "No, I'm not using any menopausal hormone therapy. I don't want to use any synthetics." Prescriptions plummeted, and that fear still lingers today. When you suggest MHT, women say, "No, no, the risks are too great."

But here's the thing, the WHI study was not representative of the women who actually want to use MHT to get through menopause. The women studied were an older, postmenopausal population. Of the more than 27,000 women enrolled, the average age was 63, and the age range spanned to 79. They also had other health risks: they were generally sedentary women who were not in a healthy weight range. The study was specifically designed to see if starting MHT later, after a woman had gone through menopause, would help reduce the risk of diseases like osteoporosis and heart disease, which otherwise would rise during this time. Not only was it not beneficial, they found, but it seemed harmful—the researchers had to stop the study early because participants were showing an increased risk of heart disease, breast cancer, stroke, and dementia. But later reviews of this study have concluded that MHT can be used safely and judiciously by many women, especially if they use it within the 10-year window surrounding menopause.

The Million Women Study recruited 1,084,110 women in the United Kingdom who were younger—perimenopausal or just at the onset of menopause—and more active and generally leaner. They found a somewhat increased risk of breast cancer. A more recent meta-analysis published in *BMJ* in 2020 suggests that increased risks of breast cancer are associated with longer-term hormone use; it also found that the risk varies depending on preparation type and declines more dramatically than previously thought once MHT is stopped.

It's also important to note that MHT has come a long way since the early 2000s. Today MHT is available in lower doses and different formulations. Different delivery methods are also available, such as transdermal estrogen, which may have a lower risk than oral hormones.

If you still have your uterus, doctors will prescribe a combination of estrogen and progesterone, since estrogen alone will thicken the lining of the uterus and create a higher risk of uterine cancer. If you have had a hysterectomy and no longer have a uterus, your doctor may prescribe estrogen only. Estrogen typically comes as a pill, patch, or gel. You also have the option of using creams, rings, or suppositories for localized use in the vagina to treat dryness and atrophy. Progesterone (or progestin, a synthetic form of the hormone) is available through an oral pill or through an IUD. You can also take combined estrogen and progesterone preparations as either an oral medication or a patch that you wear on your skin.

All these choices make it easier to target MHT to an individual's specific needs and make the treatment safer overall. We also have a better understanding of the time frame in which MHT is most effective and poses the least amount of risk.

In a research review published in 2014, researchers concluded that hormone therapy had more benefit than risk and helped control symptoms, prevent bone loss and fracture, and improve metabolic health in women younger than 60 who began using it within 10 years of their last period. This review showed that the risk of breast cancer for women who had had a hysterectomy and received estrogen-only therapy was actually reduced. The researchers concluded that "HT for most newly menopausal women is safe and effective." A 2019 review published in the journal *Womens Health (Lond)* echoed these findings. The key is starting within that 10-year window and prior to age 60.

Let's turn now to the potential benefits of MHT. We know that it's very effective for alleviating hot flashes and night sweats, which are two of the biggest complaints from women going through menopause. It also might help with vaginal dryness (local estrogen is particularly beneficial for that), mood swings, brain fog, anxiety, depression, anger, and sleeping issues, though research is ongoing.

Research shows that MHT can help preserve bone mass. Unfortunately, it's not terribly effective at preserving lean mass and reducing fat gain. It may reduce the amount of belly fat gain in some women, but not in highly active or already very physically fit women. Fortunately, exercise is good for both bone health and body composition.

MHT is not risk-free. If you're older than 60 or greater than 10 years from menopause, there's some evidence that it may increase your risk of Alzheimer's and dementia. The breast cancer risk is small, but it may increase depending on the formulation the longer you're on it. The pill form of MHT increases the risk of blood clots in both the legs and lungs. It's not a large margin, but it's not insignificant. Depending on the preparation, delivery method, and dose, MHT is linked to a minimally increased risk of stroke.

This is why you want to work with your doctor. The MHT types and forms you can use most effectively depend on many factors, including your individual risk factors, your preexisting conditions, whether you've had a hysterectomy, whether you have any specific clotting factors, your cardiovascular disease risk factors, your age, and how close to menopause you are. Your doctor can monitor you to make sure any risk factors you may have for metabolic and cardiovascular diseases are not increasing. Your doctor can also help you wean yourself off MHT when the time comes.

For more resources about MHT, you can visit the North American Menopause Society as well as the Australian Menopause Society online. Both of their websites have easy-to-understand descriptions of the different formulations, their delivery mechanism, and their risk factors, and both provide printable PDFs that you can bring to your doctor for discussion.

WHAT ABOUT ORAL CONTRACEPTIVES?

Once you're through menopause, you no longer need to worry about getting pregnant, so you no longer need to be taking "the pill." If you're taking the pill as you go into menopause, be aware that it introduces some tricky complications. Taking oral contraceptives can mask many of the symptoms of perimenopause, so it can be difficult to know where you are in your menopausal transition. In fact, adding to the confusion, if you're taking pills that have estrogen and progestin, you may continue to bleed as you would on your period, even after menopause. (This is not a period per se, as many think it is, but rather a withdrawal bleed that mimics your period.)

> Once you're in your late forties, talk to your doctor about transitioning off the pill, which increases your risk for blood clots as you age. Your doctor may advise using an IUD or progestin-only pill through these early transition years or could suggest adjusting your medications to menopausal hormone therapy instead.

ARE BIOIDENTICAL HORMONES BETTER?

Because the nervousness about synthetic hormones is so persistent, even women who are interested in MHT will sometimes shy away from traditional hormone therapy and instead want to use "bioidentical hormones," which are hormones derived from a natural source, such as wild yams, and have the same molecular structure as the body's natural hormones.

What is important to realize is that all hormones you're taking are "synthetic" because they're being derived from another source that is not a human being. The hormones from yams come from labs the same way that Premarin (conjugated estrogens) is made in a lab using urine from pregnant mares (yes, seriously). What's more, some of the FDA-regulated hormones like progesterone come from the same source as the bioidentical hormones, including yam plants.

The real issue when you go the bioidentical route is regulation. If you're interested in bioidentical hormones, I would urge you to get a prescription from your doctor, as prescribed hormones are clinically tested and regulated through federal agencies, so you know the specific dosage of hormones that you are getting.

I also caution against buying all-natural bioidentical hormones from Amazon or anywhere else online, and I'd even be wary of buying over-the-counter hormones.

The nonprescription "compounded" bioidentical hormones are created by individual pharmacies and are not regulated by a national body. You are not guaranteed a specific dosage because the delivery mechanism and the potency of the compounded product are specific to the pharmacy that created it.

Some doctors or compounding pharmacies that sell compounded therapies will offer salivary or blood tests to assess your hormone levels and create a "personalized" product. Don't believe it. At this time of your life, your hormone levels can vary from day to day or even hourly. The North American Menopause Society has supported actions of the US Congress, the FDA, and scientific organizations that have warned about the potential harm that can be done by compounded bioidentical hormones.

NONHORMONE INTERVENTIONS

Not everyone needs or wants MHT. There are other prescription medications that women can use with great success to manage some of their symptoms. Specifically, antidepressants can be really effective for relieving the mood disorders, anxiety, depression, and brain fog that can come during the menopausal transition as hormone changes disrupt the levels of your brain's chemical messengers serotonin and norepinephrine. These neurotransmitters have also been linked to depression.

So if you're seriously affected by mood disorder and brain fog, then you might want to consider using an SSRI antidepressant like citalopram (Celexa). Evidence shows that norepinephrine plays a role in the physiology of hot flashes, so antidepressants like serotonin and norepinephrine reuptake inhibitors (SNRIs like Venlafaxine) can have the added benefit of relieving hot flashes and night sweats.

Lofexidine, which traditionally has been used to treat high blood pressure (and more recently to manage opioid withdrawal), has been found to reduce hot flashes by up to 65 percent. It works by modulating and stabilizing your levels of serotonin and norepinephrine, which in turn helps stabilize your brain's response to your core temperature. Another blood pressure medication, clonidine (Catapres, Kapvay), which is typically prescribed as a pill or patch, might also provide some relief from hot flashes.

Fezolinetant, which is an oral, nonhormone therapy in clinical development to treat sex hormone–related disorders, has shown great promise for treating vasomotor symptoms like hot flashes. A recent study published in *Menopause* that included more than 350 women found that more than 80 percent of the participants taking fezolinetant enjoyed a significant reduction in symptoms; symptoms in more than half of the women taking the treatment were reduced by 90 percent or more. If and when fezolinetant will be available depends on FDA approval. But these results are promising.

One surprising alternative treatment that has gotten some mainstream media attention is gabapentin (Neurontin), which is an antiseizure medicine commonly used to treat epilepsy. Past research has shown that 1,800 milligrams a day of gabapentin can decrease the frequency and severity of hot flashes and also seems to improve sleep quality. That's a high dosage, so I don't really recommend it; gabapentin increases heart rate variability in female athletes, which can give a false sense of recovery. I would stick to antidepressants instead, if you do not have contraindications to them.

Again, these alternatives may be helpful if you're experiencing symptoms like mood swings, depression, hot flashes, and night sweats. To treat symptoms like vaginal dryness, joint pain, bone pain, or a lot of brain fog, you might be better off considering MHT, which will also help those vasomotor symptoms.

ADAPTOGENS

I am a big fan of adaptogens because, generally speaking, you can use them as long as you want at any time of life without worrisome side effects. They're beneficial for many aspects of your health and wellness, even beyond easing menopausal symptoms.

In a nutshell, adaptogens are plants that increase your body's resistance to stress. They do so by targeting your hypothalamic-pituitary-adrenal (HPA) axis, a neuroendocrine system that controls your reaction to stress and regulates various body functions, such as digestion, mood, temperature control, and immunity. When you take adaptogens, they build up in your body over time and block some of your cortisol response, so that you experience less stress. (And what woman doesn't need that, especially during midlife?) Depending on the adaptogens, they may have either a stimulating or a relaxing effect on your nervous system. They help significantly with fatigue, cognition, anxiety, and vasomotor symptoms.

Adaptogens have been around and used in traditional medicine for thousands of years. Over the past decade or so, they have received more attention from Western medical researchers, specifically the North American Menopause Society (NAMS) and the National Institutes of Health (NIH), which funds this research.

NEXT LEVEL MENOPAUSE MAKEOVER: A COMPETITIVE TRAIL RUNNER REINS IN HER RUNAWAY SYMPTOMS

CAIT,* 46, came to me feeling like a wreck after being hit by a perimenopause train. More than anything, she desperately wants her running mojo back.

GENERAL ASSESSMENT

It's the rare woman who moves through menopause without at least a few symptoms. Some unfortunate ones get blindsided by all of them. That was Cait, who at just 46 started experiencing an onslaught of menopause symptoms including hot flashes, mood changes, sudden weight gain, poor sleep, anxiety, anger, swollen breasts, lots of bloating, and lack of sex drive in the span of just three or four months. As a competitive trail runner, she had traditionally been very lean. Now she was 34 percent body fat, up from her usual 19 percent.

Everything was suffering. Her anger and anxiety were hurting her relationships and affecting her work. She would usually cope by going running, but her running was also negatively impacted, setting her up for a vicious cycle. At this point, she wanted to know if MHT could help her get her life back on track.

Her nutrition wasn't great. She was taking in lots of simple sugars during her runs, which I suspected was disrupting her gut microbiome. An unhealthy gut combined with fatigue from not sleeping left her craving and eating more carbohydrates, which combined with the increased insulin resistance that accompanies menopause, meant she was having fluctuations in blood sugar and a lot of mood swings.

Her protein intake was really low, maybe one gram per kilogram per day. That was bad for rebuilding her muscles, obviously. But it was also bad for her moods and left her more susceptible to depression, anxiety, and brain fog because she didn't have enough amino acids crossing the blood-brain barrier to help even out her neurotransmitters, like serotonin, which dip as estrogen goes haywire.

The poor sleep was definitely doing a number on her weight. Lack of sleep, especially during menopause, really decreases insulin sensitivity and increases the body's stimulus to store belly fat. Her overall stress load was really high, especially when you take into account all the symptoms she was having along with lack of sleep.

There was a lot going on here.

Because her symptoms were all-consuming and unlivable, my first recommendation was for her to discuss hormone support with her physician. This was not a case to try to use adaptogens. Adaptogens can help mitigate some symptoms and level the playing field, so to speak. But with the severity of her symptoms, MHT was in order. Her doctor agreed and she started using an estradiol patch and progesterone cream.

We needed to decrease her training load and increase her food intake. She was in a low energy availability (LEA) state, having fallen into the calories in, calories out mentality and believing that the less you eat and the more you train, the thinner you'll get. But that is not correct. We also needed to focus on some key training sessions rather than piling on training at every turn, which was keeping her cortisol elevated and doing more damage rather than helping her get on track mentally and physically.

We overhauled her diet, doubling her protein intake to 2 grams per kilogram of body weight per day and, to support her training routine, increasing her carbohydrate intake to 2.5 to 3 grams per kilogram per day, focusing on fruits and vegetables, especially cruciferous vegetables like cabbage and cauliflower, as her primary sources to help get more healthy bacteria in her gut and to help moderate her hormonal fluctuation. I suggested she eat fermented food every day to further bolster her gut health.

Instead of using gels for all her long runs, we had her fuel properly beforehand and take some protein/carbohydrate bites with her for fuel. I wanted to really decrease levels of the bacteria in her gut that were feeding off of and craving the simple sugars.

We also really needed to help her get some sleep. That meant establishing pre-bedtime habits to activate her parasympathetic drive as much as possible to improve sleep. She cooled the room temperature in her bedroom, shut off screens before bed, added white noise, and had cold tart cherry juice 30 minutes before bedtime.

HER NEW ROUTINE

Here's how her new schedule looks after our makeover. Because her situation was so severe, we made these changes in a stepwise fashion. We significantly dialed back her training at first and then added more back three weeks in.

MONDAY: 11:30 a.m. open water swim, no tempo run. Open water swimming is quiet and relaxing and has a parasympathetic drive. So we keep the swims in her schedule.

After 3 weeks: Add a 20-minute easy jog after the swim.

TUESDAY: 6:30 a.m. very easy 40-minute trail run, with a snack before and breakfast immediately after. This lets her sleep in and get in a nice run that isn't as taxing.

After 3 weeks: 6 a.m. very easy 60-minute trail run. Evening yoga session in her house to activate her parasympathetic response.

WEDNESDAY: Lunch PT session as usual. Splitting lunch before and after to prevent her from becoming catabolic.

THURSDAY: Sleep in, no trail run in the morning. 6 p.m. easy 25 to 30 minute trail run just for the joy of it. No intervals. Dinner immediately after.

After 3 weeks: Increase the intensity of the evening run to a rating of perceived exertion (RPE) of 7 (max).

FRIDAY: 11:30 a.m. open water swim, same as Monday.

SATURDAY: 90 to 120 minute hike in the hills, maintaining an RPE of 5 to 6 on a 1 to 10 scale.

After 3 weeks: Increase the intensity to a hike/jog, going to 7 or 8 RPE on the inclines.

SUNDAY: Hot yoga or whatever chill activity she feels like.

At the end of three weeks, she felt really relaxed, had been sleeping better, felt less stressed, and her moods were more positive and in control. So we increased her intensity on a few of the sessions and maintained that schedule for 10 months.

THE RESULTS

Cait lost 14 pounds and reduced her body fat percentage 10 points to 24 percent. Our next step is to add heavy lifting into her schedule, which will help improve lean mass and strength on the trail. She settled on a Climara patch and a Mirena IUD for her MHT. She also started using a Whoop band so she could track her quality and quantity of sleep.

Most importantly, she's enjoying running again. Her stress is lower, so she can train hard on hard days and recover well when she backs off and goes easy on the easy days. She's rediscovered her love for the sport and has her mojo back.

What follows are descriptions of the adaptogens that I have personally found most useful, along with the ones that the women in my practice have had success with. Some are stimulating and some are calming, so consider those effects when determining what time of day to use them. Choose one based on your most severe symptoms and start there. After two weeks, if you feel you need additional help, try adding a second. Remember, less is more when it comes to adaptogens. And as with any new therapy, check with your doctor if you have concerns about drug or other therapy interactions.

ASHWAGANDHA (CALMING)

MAIN FUNCTION: Acting as a hormonal precursor, increases luteinizing hormone (T3, T4)

Native to India and North Africa, ashwagandha increases your dehydro-epiandrosterone (DHEA) testosterone, thereby reducing cortisol and lowering anxiety and depression. This one is a relaxant, but in an energized-but-chill way. It helps to preserve brain health and protect against cognitive impairment, so it is very good at clearing out the brain fog.

Ashwagandha is especially good for reducing stress and anxiety. In a 2019 study, researchers found that stressed-out adults taking 250 to 600 milligrams of ashwagandha a day for eight weeks enjoyed a significant reduction in their serum cortisol and stress levels as well as marked improvement in their sleep quality. Another study published the same year echoed those findings, showing that as little as 240 milligrams a day lowered levels of anxiety and stress as well as levels of morning cortisol in a group of adults who struggled with stress.

Some studies show that ashwagandha helps regulate your blood lipids, specifically reducing your total cholesterol as well as your less desirable low-density lipoproteins, or LDL cholesterol. It also supports your thyroid, which is good for women during this time, as low levels of thyroid hormones can worsen symptoms of menopause. Ashwagandha may also help regulate your body temperature to reduce hot flashes.

As an anti-inflammatory, ashwagandha is extremely helpful during menopause, when systemic inflammation levels can rise and lead to soreness, poor recovery, and susceptibility to disease. It also may reduce delayed onset muscle soreness (DOMS) after a hard workout.

Because it lowers cortisol, ashwagandha helps with insulin sensitivity and blood sugar control, making you less inclined to store fat. So it may help you maintain and improve your body composition and reduce abdominal fat. Research on athletes shows that it may improve strength and endurance.

DOSE: Ascribing to "less is more," start with the smallest effective dose, then slowly increase if you are not finding results. Take 300 milligrams twice a day for menopausal symptoms, body composition benefits, and blood glucose control (taken for at least two months).

SMALLEST EFFECTIVE DOSE: 250 milligrams a day for stress reduction and anti-inflammatory benefits. Look for ashwagandha supplements that contain withanolides, saponins, and alkaloids (from the root), with a withanolide concentration of 5 to 8 percent. Ashwagandha works well with black pepper to improve absorption or with Holy Basil in the afternoon for calming effects and better sleep (not as a sedative, but by modulating neurotransmitters and cortisol).

CAUTION: Ashwagandha affects your T3 and T4 thyroid hormones, so it may help with hypothyroidism. If you're on thyroid medications, however, you should not take this adaptogen. Men with (or a history of) hormone-sensitive prostate cancer should not use ashwagandha.

HOLY BASIL (CALMING)

MAIN FUNCTION: Anxiety and stress reduction

Known in the Hindi language as *tulsi*, Holy Basil is not like the seasoning you toss in your Sunday marinara sauce. Probably because of its ability to combat stress, improve blood sugar control, act as an antioxidant, and enhance immunity as well as reduce anxiety, depression, and poor sleep, it's revered in traditional medicine for its ability to promote a healthy mind, body, and spirit.

Holy Basil is so broadly beneficial for metabolic health that a 2017 review of 24 studies concluded that it "is an effective treatment for lifestyle-related chronic diseases including diabetes, metabolic syndrome, and psychological stress."

SMALLEST EFFECTIVE DOSE: 500 milligrams, twice a day. If you'd like to pair Holy Basil with ashwagandha for anxiety reduction and sleep, start with Holy Basil and use for three weeks. Then add ashwagandha, if needed.

CAUTION: Holy Basil reduces blood-clotting capacity. Do not use if you are on anti-coagulants.

RHODIOLA ROSEA (STIMULATING)

MAIN FUNCTION: Combating fatigue and improving cognitive function

Rhodiola, also known as "golden root," is a natural stimulant that helps balance your levels of neurotransmitters like serotonin, norepinephrine, and dopamine. During the menopausal years, these chemicals can get out of balance, causing mood swings and anxiety and contributing to hot flashes. Taking rhodiola can improve concentration, reduce mental fatigue, decrease anxiety and irritability, and decrease the frequency and severity of hot flashes.

Rhodiola is a selective estrogen reuptake modulator (SERM), so it may prevent, delay, or mitigate menopause-related cognitive, psychological, cardiovascular, and osteoporotic (bone-thinning) conditions.

By normalizing the release of your stress hormones, particularly cortisol, rhodiola improves your mood and fights fatigue. It also helps balance melatonin and serotonin, which contributes to reducing fatigue (and ironically, can help highly stressed individuals have a great sleep!). It also improves your energy metabolism by boosting your mitochondria function, so you can produce more ATP (adenosine triphosphate), which provides the energy your muscles use to contract more quickly. Athletes of all sexes and ages benefit from rhodiola to elevate exercise performance.

Research suggests that rhodiola may also promote neurogenesis—the formation of new brain cells. That's good news for menopausal women, who are losing the brain-protecting benefits of progesterone. Though more research is needed, a 2012 study found that rhodiola may be helpful at alleviating brain fog and mental fatigue. Another study from the same year found that 400 milligrams of rhodiola per day significantly improved participants' symptoms of stress starting in as little as three days.

From a psychological standpoint, taking rhodiola improves concentration, decreases irritability, lowers anxiety, and gives you your mojo back, all within the first week of usage. If you're looking for one adaptogen to try, I would recommend starting with rhodiola and see how it helps with your symptoms before adding any others.

DOSE: 150 to 600 milligrams a day.

SMALLEST EFFECTIVE DOSE: 150 milligrams, twice a day. Rhodiola goes well with schisandra, but if you're going to pair them, start with schisandra, then add rhodiola after two weeks.

CAUTION: It's best to take rhodiola early in the day because it's a bit of a stimulant (although as mentioned above, it works on melatonin and serotonin, so some people experience sleepiness). Though it is generally very safe, there is some evidence that rhodiola may lower blood pressure. That's generally a benefit but can be problematic for women who already have low blood pressure or are taking blood pressure medications like ACE inhibitors. Do not take rhodiola if you're on immunosuppressants or prescription monoamine oxidase inhibitors (MAOIs), which is a class of antidepressants. Because rhodiola rosea root can have such strong estrogenic effects, it would be wise to avoid it if estrogen is contraindicated for you.

SCHISANDRA (STIMULATING)

MAIN FUNCTION: Boosting endurance, mental performance, and working capacity

Also known as five-flavored-fruit, schisandra (Magnolia berry) is widely used in traditional Chinese medicine. It stimulates your central nervous system, improves cognition, and balances the neurotransmitters, like serotonin and dopamine, that can get out of whack during menopause. It also improves your energy levels and clears out the brain fog that can come during the menopausal years, giving you calm energy and focus.

Schisandra is a phytoestrogen, so it acts like a weak form of estrogen in your body. That means it helps modulate the estrogen fluctuations that are common in the transition to menopause. This makes it a good adaptogen for reducing the frequency and severity of hot flashes.

In a 2016 study of women between the ages of 40 and 70 who suffered with high levels of menopausal symptoms such as low mood, insomnia, palpitations, and hot flashes, taking schisandra significantly improved their symptoms (especially hot flashes, sweating, and heart palpitations).

Schisandra can also help with your fitness and endurance. It increases blood vessel compliance (due to its phytoestrogen properties) and strengthens your mitochondria (where your cells make energy), so it improves your exercise capacity. It may also improve your strength, according to a 2020 study of 45 healthy postmenopausal women with an average age of 62. These researchers found that women given 1,000 milligrams of schisandra a day saw gains in their quadriceps muscle strength and had lower lactate levels at rest (a marker associated with muscle fatigue) than participants who took a placebo over the same 12-week period.

DOSE: 500 milligrams to 2 grams daily of schisandra extract or 1.5 to 6 grams of crude schisandra daily. (The powder has a bitter nutty flavor that goes well in coffee.)

SMALLEST EFFECTIVE DOSE FOR MENOPAUSE SYMPTOMS: 13.5 milligrams per kilogram per day (for example, 830 milligrams for a 140-pound woman). Schisandra goes well with rhodiola, but take schisandra (which has a milder estrogenic effect) on its own first for two weeks, then add rhodiola if desired.

CAUTION: Avoid taking schisandra late in the afternoon or evening, as it has a caffeine-like effect on alertness and could disrupt your sleep. It can cause heartburn or upset stomach in some people.

MACA (STIMULATING)

MAIN FUNCTION: Sex hormone support

Sometimes referred to as Peruvian ginseng, maca root is a hormone modulator and strong anti-inflammatory that regulates adrenal and thyroid function and also works as a steroid hormone—so it's pretty powerful. If you're looking for one "all-around" adaptogen to try, maca is a good one.

Research finds that maca can improve both mood and energy levels, alleviate brain fog, and dramatically decrease the feelings of anxiety and depression that are common during the menopausal years. Some users describe it as giving them a natural high. If you're struggling to get your mojo back, maca can definitely help.

When used early in perimenopause, research indicates that maca can be as effective as MHT for counteracting vasomotor symptoms like hot flashes and night sweats. By helping to regulate adrenal and thyroid function, it also improves energy and fights fatigue.

Maca has been popular among bodybuilders and athletes for years because of claims that it helps build muscle, enhances endurance performance, and increases strength. More research is needed to verify all those claims. There is also some evidence that it might help with sexual dysfunction in postmenopausal women who use antidepressants.

SMALLEST EFFECTIVE DOSE: 2.0 grams per day for vasomotor and hormonal symptoms, or 3.5 grams per day for mood and psychological benefits.

CAUTION: Because it regulates adrenal and thyroid function (it contains goitrogens), don't use maca if you're on thyroid medication. Some of the products that contain maca are also on the WADA (World Anti-Doping Agency) banned substances list. So if you're a drug-tested athlete, it's probably best to not use this one.

FAQS ON ADAPTOGENS

Can you use more than one adaptogen? What should you look for when buying an adaptogen? How long do they take to work? Here are the answers to the most commonly asked questions regarding adaptogens.

CAN YOU COMBINE ADAPTOGENS?

Yes, you definitely can. I generally advise people to consider what they want to use them for. What are your main symptoms? Are you having major hot flashes? Are you having mostly brain fog? Are you fatigued? Are you unable to work out at your maximum capacity? Consider your most severe symptoms and choose the adaptogen that is best suited to alleviate them. Take it for the recommended two weeks to see how it is working. Then you can add others as needed for secondary symptoms. There is no harm in combining adaptogens. Most people do. But you also might find that adding one gives you no additional benefit, in which case there's no point in continuing with it. Taking ashwagandha is what most women start with for general symptoms.

WHAT SHOULD I LOOK FOR WHEN BUYING ADAPTOGENS?

Because these are plant compounds, purity is definitely a priority. You want to find a reliable, reputable, organic source. So check the label to make sure that the adaptogen is certified organic. The dosage should be clearly spelled out on the label, so you know exactly how much of the active ingredient you are taking.

IS THERE A DANGER OF BEING ON ADAPTOGENS TOO LONG?

Adaptogens build up in your system over time, so there's generally a benefit to sustained use. That said, you may eventually develop a tolerance to them, so it is a good idea to cycle them. When you first start taking adaptogens, use them six or seven weeks and then take a few days off before starting up again. Once you've been on them for a while, you can shorten the cycle and take them for a cycle of three weeks on and two days off to prevent building up a tolerance or developing side effects.

DOES IT MATTER WHAT FORM I USE?

Nope. If you're someone who likes powders, you can use them in smoothies. If you prefer tablets or capsules, those work just as well. If you like tinctures, add it to your tea. Choose whatever is going to fit best in your life.

CAN I USE ADAPTOGENS PREEMPTIVELY BEFORE I GET SYMPTOMS?

Yes, definitely. Adaptogens are all about downgrading our stress. That's good for everybody from younger athletes to postmenopausal women. You don't have to be experiencing symptoms to enjoy benefits. And they can help you avoid some symptoms down the road.

CAN I USE ADAPTOGENS IF I'M ALREADY USING MHT?

Yes, but with a caveat. MHT is prescribed for symptoms, to help you get through the menopause transition. If you are still having symptoms, which ones are you still experiencing? Are you still having brain fog? Are you still having trouble falling asleep? List your symptoms and match them up with the adaptogens that address them and then add them to your menopause symptom arsenal. Some women ask if they can use adaptogens instead of MHT. If you're already on MHT and want to switch to adaptogens, I recommend working with your physician to slowly taper off of MHT to see which symptoms come back. Then you can choose adaptogens to mitigate those symptoms.

5

KICK UP YOUR CARDIO

At this point in your life, society is telling you to slow down. Training the way you always have just might make you do that—whether you like it or not.

"Slow down."

"Take it easy."

"You don't want to hurt yourself."

How many times have you heard those messages? That's what society tells people when they get older. Older men have some role models like Tom Brady (who, at age 43, had played in a record-setting 10 Super Bowls), Tiger Woods (45), and Laird Hamilton (57) showing them that they don't need to slow down after 40 or 50—nor *should* they. But there just aren't as many women paving the way . . . yet.

A few women pioneers have blazed the way before us. Kathrine Switzer, the first woman to officially run the Boston Marathon in 1967 despite a *lot* of pushback (literally—officials tried to push her off the course), ran Boston again in 2017 at age 70, and only about 24 minutes slower than when she first ran it. She remains one of running's most iconic figures. Olympic swimming sensation Dara Torres was the oldest swimmer to compete in the Olympics at 41, and she went on to add boxing and Barre to her swimming regimen to keep fit into her late forties. Fifty-three-year-old cyclist Rebecca Rusch, a world champion multiple times, is still crushing the competition on her mountain bike, most recently winning the 350-mile Iditarod Trail Invitational. And world kickboxing champ, former Israeli Commando instructor, and ultra-endurance cyclist Leah Goldstein beat everyone—including the men—in the 2021 Race Across America at the age of 52.

These women athletes are emblematic of our generation—we are the first to do things differently and to want to *keep* doing things differently. We want to keep lining up for 10Ks and triathlons and joining our friends for the CrossFit WOD. That means we can't do what generations before us have done—we can't slow down. In fact, we need to do the exact opposite. We need to sprint.

Yes, sprint. No matter if you're an endurance athlete or someone who works out for the mental and physical benefits, you'll reap many more rewards from your exercise time by turning up the intensity (and turning down the volume) a couple of times a week. (And then *truly* recovering on other days—something too few of us do!)

Research dating back to the early to mid-2000s confirms that sprint training is good for every type of active person. In her groundbreaking study published in *Journal of Applied Physiology* in 2005, exercise scientist Kirsten Burgomaster showed that two weeks of regular sprint interval training (SIT) didn't just make the study participants better sprinters, but also improved their endurance—doubling their time to fatigue.

Since then, dozens more studies have solidified the conclusion that interval training is the fastest way to improve nearly all aspects of performance, including improved insulin sensitivity and ability to use oxygen, which enables you to burn more fat and get more fuel into your working muscles. Though much of the early research was done on sedentary men, numerous studies in recent years have shown how well high exercise intensity works for menopausal women.

One such study published in *Menopause* reported that two weeks of high-intensity interval training (HIIT) sessions consisting of 10 one-minute cycling efforts at peak power separated by one minute of active recovery, three times a week (including a warm-up and cool-down), improved cardiovascular function as well as pedaling along at moderate intensity (65 percent of peak power) for 40 minutes three times a week for two weeks.

Even if you run marathons, including ultras, dialing down the volume and turning up the intensity once you hit menopause will help you run longer and stronger. Remember, as a woman, you're already built for endurance. If you've been an endurance athlete for most of your younger life, you have *plenty* of miles in your legs at this point. What you need to do to stay strong in the game is not piling on more miles, but making more of those miles count.

WHY SIT IS THE BEST FORM OF HIIT FOR MENOPAUSE

For menopausal women, high-intensity sprint interval training sessions can provide the metabolic stimulus to trigger the performance-boosting body composition changes that our hormones helped us achieve in our premenopausal years.

The key here is the intensity. In high-intensity interval training, alternating short bursts of *hard* exercise are followed by relatively short recovery periods. So if you're using heart rate as a guide, anything that sends your heart rate above about 85 percent of your maximum is high intensity. When you reach your menopausal years, it's very important to incorporate the shortest, sharpest form of HIIT: sprint interval training. As the term indicates, SIT sessions include super-short, 10- to 30-second sprint-style efforts. They are extremely beneficial for both peri- and postmenopausal women.

One of the biggest benefits of SIT training is improvement in body composition. SIT training increases lean muscle mass and reduces fat mass in a relatively short period of time. In a 2019 study published in *Medicine & Science in Sports & Exercise*, researchers had a group of postmenopausal women, ages 47 to 59, perform 20-minute bouts of SIT—alternating eight seconds of sprinting on a stationary bike at about 85 percent of their maximum heart rate with 12 seconds of easy pedaling—three times a week for eight weeks. By study's end, the women had lost fat, regained lean muscle mass, and improved their aerobic fitness by 12 percent after what amounted to only eight hours of actual exercise over eight weeks' time.

In another study, researchers had a group of older postmenopausal women with type 2 diabetes, average age of 69, either perform the same type of SIT training—alternating eight seconds of sprinting on a stationary bike with 12 seconds of easy pedaling, twice a week for 16 weeks—or perform 40 minutes of moderate-intensity cycling twice a week for the same period. While both groups gained muscle and lost fat, only the SIT training women shed stubborn belly fat. The sprinters lost more than 8 percent of total abdominal fat and 24 percent of visceral (the deep, health-wrecking) abdominal fat—all without changing anything in their diet.

SIT helps burn off belly fat and improve body composition on a couple of fronts. For one, it coaxes your body into burning more fat for energy when you're not exercising. As you reach perimenopause, your body burns less fat at rest and stores more of it. SIT turns that around. This type of high-intensity work demands carbohydrates and pulls a lot of glucose from your bloodstream. (Premenopause, E2 helped with this blood sugar control; now you need high-intensity training to get the job done well.) Your body responds by replenishing your muscle and liver glycogen (carbohydrate) stores with carbohydrate and using more of your fat while you're at rest, because it knows that you're going to need those muscle stores to perform those intense exercise bouts again.

SIT training strengthens and increases the amount of your energy-producing mitochondria, improves insulin sensitivity, and lowers fasting blood sugar levels, all of which is good for your overall cardiovascular and metabolic health. Your mitochondria tend to become less functional over time—regardless of menopause—and HIIT training can help keep them running on all cylinders. A Mayo Clinic study published in *Cell Metabolism* found that the mitochondrial function of older exercisers (ages 65 to 80) soared 69 percent after 12 weeks of regular HIIT training. The older exercisers, both male and female, saw no mitochondrial gains following lower-intensity programs.

HIGH INTENSITY FOR ENDURANCE

Just as heavy strength training can benefit endurance athletes, so can sprint training. Research shows that, depending on how fit you are when you start, infusing your regular endurance routine with high-intensity efforts can boost your VO_2 max (how much oxygen you can use) by as much as 46 percent, increase your stroke volume (how much blood your heart pumps out per beat), raise your power at lactate threshold, and significantly lower your resting heart rate. SIT also increases your mitochondria content. All of these improvements enable you to stay "aerobic" longer so that you can burn more fat at higher-intensity exercise. Remember, too, that SIT helps postmenopausal women regain some lean body mass, which they need for producing power in endurance sports.

Even though SIT is super-hard and your legs (and brain) may be screaming for you to stop, it is a fantastic stress-reducer (once you're done, that is!). That's good not only for your mental health but also for your physical health, including reducing abdominal fat.

Remember, levels of your stress hormone, cortisol, rise during menopause. That sets you up for a vicious cycle of storing belly fat, which produces more inflammation and stress. In fact, deep belly fat has about four times as many cortisol receptors as the regular fat that sits under your skin. So not only does deep belly fat trigger more cortisol production, but it also leads to more belly fat storage. SIT breaks this cycle.

When you do SIT, your body pumps out more human growth hormone (HGH), increases testosterone, decreases estrone (the less desirable form of estrogen produced by fat tissue), and counteracts cortisol. The result is a reduction of cortisol and lower stress levels overall. With less cortisol, you have less stimulus for putting on body fat. With more HGH and testosterone (both of which are anabolic, or muscle-making), you have an increased stimulus for putting on lean muscle. When you follow up that SIT session with some protein (see chapter 10 for more nutrition advice), you'll really maximize those body composition changes.

This is the opposite of the metabolic chain of events that happens after long, steady endurance exercise. I'm not telling anyone they should give up their two- to three-hour runs or three- to four-hour bike rides (or whatever endurance you love to do!). There's a time and a place for those. But long endurance exercise actually stimulates an increase in cortisol that tends to linger. Researchers who tested hair samples from endurance athletes found a correlation between cortisol levels in their hair and their endurance training volume. You need to balance out endurance training with short, sharp, high-intensity training.

SIT also triggers an anti-inflammatory response: when you do it regularly over time, you have lower total levels of inflammation. That's important because, as you know, inflammation, like cortisol, rises as our sex hormones fluctuate and decline. With less inflammation, your body recovers better. It also absorbs iron better, which is important for menopausal women, who sometimes become anemic and don't understand why (it's the inflammation). In that way, SIT helps with general health as well as performance.

Sometimes women worry that pushing themselves too hard will compromise their immunity and leave them vulnerable to getting sick. The opposite is actually true. In a 2018 study titled "Debunking the Myth of Exercise-Induced Immune Suppression," researchers from the United Kingdom explained that when people start exercising hard, their "natural killer cells," which fight infection, increase by up to tenfold. Then a funny thing happens—when they're done with their high-intensity session, the immune cell levels in their bloodstream plummet for a couple of hours. This is why some observers have long thought that hard exercise makes a person more vulnerable to infection. But those immune cells haven't been destroyed. Instead, they have been deployed to areas that are more likely to become infected, like your gut and lungs. They're just on high alert!

When you push your body into the red, you also stimulate what is known as vascular endothelial growth factor, which makes your blood vessels more responsive. That improves both performance and blood pressure, increases your overall cardiovascular health, and reduces hot flashes. Your body will be able to respond to exercise demands more quickly and to tolerate hot and cold because your blood vessels can react more readily when you need to send blood to the skin or the core to cool down or warm up. Again, before menopause, estrogen was the main driver of healthy blood vessel function. Once it starts dwindling, you need to step in and do some of the work it used to do.

Finally, SIT training can make you smarter. As you'll recall, brain-derived neurotrophic factor (BDNF), which is responsible for brain tissue health, decreases with a lack of estrogen and with age. Know what pumps it back up? You guessed it—exercise, and high-intensity workouts in particular. The sharp, strong stimulation from a SIT session triggers an increase in BDNF along with other chemical messengers in the brain to enhance your brain remodeling, keep your gray matter healthy, and improve cognition and working memory, both of which can suffer during the menopausal years.

HOW TO DO SIT

The key to SIT is not overdoing it. High-intensity training is strong medicine. The right dose works wonders; too much can backfire and have ill effects.

During your off-season, when you're not out running, riding, hiking, or doing big events, you can do up to three SIT workouts a week, so long as you allow your body ample recovery time to bounce back from week to week. Generally speaking, however, two sessions a week are enough. During months when you're busy with lots of activity and going hard on the weekends, you can dial it back to one session a week to stay sharp.

Pick the type of exercise that works best for you. If you're not a runner, you obviously don't want to hit the track and start sprinting out of the gate! In fact, some research suggests that, in postmenopausal women, high-intensity cycling sessions are more effective than running, probably because it's easier to hit those really high intensities while cycling, without putting undue strain on your muscles and connective tissues.

There are many ways to do sprint intervals. Here are a couple of the most popular types. Always warm up thoroughly for at least 10 to 15 minutes before starting and cool down for a couple of minutes when you're done.

TABATAS

Named for the Japanese scientist Dr. Izumi Tabata, who developed these workouts, Tabata efforts are super-short and simple to do on nearly any piece of exercise equipment.

DO IT: Push as hard as possible for 20 seconds. Go super-easy for 10 seconds. Repeat six to eight times. Recover for four to five minutes with a super-easy activity. Repeat another set. Work up to three sets.

40/20s

Basically double-Tabatas, 40/20s are still short and sharp, but long enough that you can settle in and push, which builds mental and physical endurance. (Forty seconds is about the maximum I'd recommend for a SIT session.)

DO IT: Push as hard as you can for 40 seconds. Recover with a super-easy effort for 20 seconds. Repeat 10 times. Recover fully for five minutes. Repeat for another set. Work up to three sets.

30 ON 30 OFF

These SIT intervals increase the challenge by shortening the recovery time, so you're pushing and recovering for equal amounts of time.

DO IT: Push your effort as hard as you can go for 30 seconds. Go super-easy for 30 seconds. Repeat four to six times. Recover fully for four minutes. Repeat for another set. Work up to three sets.

HILL REPEATS

One easy—and incredibly effective—way to sneak in some SIT is to do hill repeats. Just go to a short hill and charge up it for 20 or 30 seconds and then walk or shuffle back down. This is a favorite of ultra-running icon Magda Boulet, who told Selene (on the menopause performance podcast *Hit Play Not Pause*) that when she's training for a big event, she'll do 20- to 30-second hill repeats because it's great training stimulation but not as hard on the body as straight-up speed work on the track.

KETTLEBELL SIT

If you're not inclined to run, swim, cycle, or do other straight-up endurance-style exercise, you can get your SIT training with kettlebells. You can simply do kettlebell swings or other full-body exercises using a Tabata regimen of going at it hard for 20 seconds, then resting for 10 seconds, for three to four rounds, recover, and then repeat as you would on a treadmill or exercise bike. Research shows these kettlebell efforts work as well as more traditional sprint training and may be more attractive and sustainable for some exercisers.

At this point, you may be wondering, *How do I fit this in with my longer endurance activity?* Don't worry, chapter 19 offers sample training schedules that will take care of that. But in general, if you've been doing lots of long, slow, or "comfortably hard" endurance sessions, you'll be substituting a SIT workout for some of those, then doing one truly long endurance session per week. (For some women, every 10 days is enough.)

HOW HARD IS HARD?

If you use a heart rate monitor or a device like a power meter on your bike, you can easily tell how hard you're going. If not, you can just go by feel. The beauty of SIT-style HIIT training is its simplicity—the goal is just to go as hard as you can, since you're only doing it for a super-short burst, so you don't actually need to watch any numbers to know that you're going "hard enough." The following chart shows what basic training zones look like. Aim your efforts at a 9 to 10, and your recovery bouts at a 2 to 3, on the RPE (rating of perceived exertion) scale.

Zone 1: Light and relaxed breathing—barely above normal. RPE 1 to 2.

Zone 2: Deep, steady, relaxed breathing. That's your aerobic, endurance-training zone. It's an RPE of 3 to 4.

Zone 3: Slightly labored. This is a steady "tempo" pace, where you're working just a bit above your endurance comfort zone. It's where you'd be if you were riding with someone just slightly faster than you. It's an RPE of 5 to 6.

Zone 4: Short, quick rhythmic breathing. This is your lactate threshold zone, right where you're hitting your sustainable upper limits. Also known as "race pace," it's an RPE of 6 to 8.

Zone 5: Hard, heavy-breath breathing. This is your VO_2 max training zone, or the top of your limits, as hard as you can go. It's an RPE of 9 to 10.

6

NOW'S THE TIME
TO LIFT HEAVY SH*T!

*Menopause demands a different
approach to strength training.*

If you do nothing else, do this: lift heavy sh*t! Muscle is your engine. It determines how fast you can run, how easily you can carry luggage, portage a kayak, climb mountains, and live a strong, active life. It gives you energy. It's also very easy to lose, especially once you hit the menopause transition.

The fact is, everyone—both men and women—naturally loses muscle and strength with age. If you do nothing to stem that loss, you can expect to lose up to 8 percent of your strength each decade after your thirtieth birthday, and that decline accelerates after age 60. So by the time you're 55, you might be 20 percent weaker. The years around menopause can make this worse, as estrogen is essential for muscle stem cell function and maintenance and is also the main driver of muscle mass and strength.

Scientists see this decline as clear as day in muscle cell studies. When researchers take estrogen away from animals, their ability to regenerate muscle stem cells (also called satellite cells) can plummet 30 to 60 percent. Likewise, when researchers take muscle biopsies in women shortly before and after their transition to menopause, they see the same thing. The number of satellite cells strongly correlates with changes in estrogen levels. That's why you might look in the mirror one day and feel like the reflection staring back is radically different from what you remember. It is.

It does not have to be that way. While everyone will lose some strength and muscle over time, you most definitely can put muscle back on and retain more of it through properly performed resistance training. And the most effective way to do this, I like to say, is to "lift heavy sh*t."

WHY YOU NEED TO LIFT HEAVY

There's a tendency for women to lift lighter weights for high repetitions, like picking up five-pound dumbbells and lifting them 20 times. This is often called "body sculpting" by trainers, who promise women that they can "tone up" without "getting bulky muscles." This mindset needs to go because it's misleading, misguided, and honestly not helpful for women whose sex hormones, lean muscle mass, and strength are on a precipitous decline. This type of lifting will build muscle endurance, but that's not what you're looking for at this stage of the game. You need muscle strength.

The other common approach is lifting in the moderate 10- to 12-repetition range. When you lift in this range, you create tiny tears in your muscle fibers, which your body repairs and fills with more material to make your muscles bigger, a process known as hypertrophy. This type of lifting can increase the amount of lean muscle mass you have, which isn't a bad thing per se. But it won't really stimulate those satellite cells and replace the muscle and strength-building stimulus that you're losing as estrogen declines. It won't make you as strong as you could be.

Building true strength is a matter of increasing the maximum force your muscle can produce in a single contraction—how much you can lift or move in one shot.

To improve that, you need to lift heavy enough to send a message to your brain that you have serious work to do and that you need all the muscle fibers possible at your disposal. You're looking to get those nerves firing and establishing those neuromuscular connections so that more of your muscle fibers will work together to create a really strong contraction and produce explosive power.

Heavy lifting is also just good for your health. Some of the most important benefits include:

INCREASED METABOLIC RATE: Heavy lifting increases your metabolic rate, or metabolism, because you're waking up more muscle fibers and muscle is very active tissue. It requires a lot of energy just to exist. When you increase your metabolic rate, you increase the number of calories you're using at rest, or your resting metabolic rate—the calories we burn just to live—which declines once we reach our sixties. So this also helps counter some of the detrimental metabolic effects that come with age.

Interestingly, lifting heavy sh*t and restoring lost muscle mass can help you burn more fat *while* you exercise. A study published in the *American Journal of Physiology—Endocrinology and Metabolism* reported that when a group of pre- and postmenopausal women pedaled a stationary bike for 45 minutes, the postmenopausal women had 33 percent lower fat burning and 19 percent less energy expenditure during the cardio bout compared to premenopausal women. Their muscle mass was also nearly nine and a half pounds lower than the muscle mass of the premenopausal women. When the scientists took that lean body mass difference into consideration, the difference in fat burning was 23 percent, with no difference in total calories burned during exercise. The researchers concluded that "LBM [lean body mass] seems to be the most important contributor to the observed changes in metabolism in women in early stages after menopause."

IMPROVED POSTURE AND STABILITY: Joint strength and stability become an issue with age, and especially with the onset of menopause, when many women start experiencing joint pain and instability for the first time. As mentioned in chapter 3, this happens during perimenopause because you have higher levels of inflammation and you're losing a bit of the strength and tension in your tendons that your sex hormones provide. By lifting heavy weights, you are stimulating your tendons to increase their tension, which will give you better overall stability in your joints and increase the ability of your muscles to support those joints when you're doing hard work. This is also true of muscles that you are not working directly, like those that stabilize and support your spine, which typically start to degrade with age. You put all those muscles to work when you lift heavy sh*t and are rewarded with better posture and healthier, stronger muscles from head to toe.

STRONGER BONES: Heavy resistance training is very good for remodeling your bones and improving bone mineral density. Research shows that resistance training is especially beneficial for strengthening cortical bone, which is the dense outer surface of bone that makes up nearly 80 percent of your skeleton.

BETTER BLOOD PRESSURE CONTROL: Heavy lifting improves your cardiovascular health. For years, the conventional wisdom was that you lift for your muscles and do cardio for your heart. But resistance training is good for your heart too. It increases your vascular compliance (your blood vessels dilating and constricting more readily), giving you better blood pressure control, better blood flow to and from your muscles, and better blood flow to and from your skin. Improvements in vascular control are important during menopause because as estrogen declines, your risk for cardiovascular disease goes up. These improvements can also help with hot flashes.

MAINTENANCE OF HEALTHY BODY COMPOSITION: Lifting heavy sh*t helps you with maintaining lean muscle and reduces fat gain. Remember, as estrogen declines, so does our anabolic (muscle-building) stimulus, and we start storing fat more easily, especially in our abdominal area. By lifting heavy sh*t, you send your muscles an anabolic signal that says, "Hey, we need to be strong to overcome this stress." This not only stimulates lean mass development but also signals to your body to decrease central and total body fat. Heavy resistance training is much more effective for changing body composition than endurance-based lifting or your typical cardiovascular exercise, especially in the years leading up to menopause and the years that follow it.

FEWER SICK DAYS: Heavy lifting even improves your immunity. Strength training creates a cascade of small proteins called cytokines that control the growth and activity of immune cells. Over the long term this effect reduces inflammation and bolsters your immune system.

So if you've always lifted in the 10-to-12 or 15-to-20 repetition range, it's time to change that up. Drop those reps into the three-to-six range and lift heavier weights to improve your muscle integrity, build strength, and be healthier through menopause and beyond.

LIGHT LIFTING IS INEFFECTIVE FOR ENDURANCE ATHLETES

Maybe you're reading this chapter and you're *so close* to being persuaded to heft some heavier weights. But a nagging voice in the back of your head says, *That's not how runners* (or cyclists or swimmers or other endurance athletes) *are supposed to lift.*

You're not alone. That "endurance" style of lifting became popular in the late 1990s and early 2000s and has stuck around to this day. But it doesn't work. The latest study to show its ineffectiveness was published in 2021 in the *European Journal of Sport Science*.

A team of researchers divided 38 marathon runners into one of three strength training groups: a heavy strength training group, who lifted heavy weights with low reps; a complex strength training group, who paired heavy strength training with plyometrics; and an endurance strength training group, who lifted light weights for high reps. For six weeks, all three groups strength-trained twice a week in addition to their normal running.

In the end, the heavy and complex trainers enjoyed significant improvements in maximum strength, running economy, and velocity at VO_2 max, while the endurance training group did not.

It's hard enough for busy women to cram in time to do all the training they want and need to do. Make it count: lift heavy sh*t.

HOW TO LIFT HEAVY SH*T

Heavy lifting is defined as lifting six reps or less with as much weight as possible. It's obviously not something that you jump straight into without building up to it, especially if you're new to resistance training.

A little goes a long way! You should not be lifting heavy for every single exercise. Instead, you want to reserve lifting heavy sh*t (LHS) for big, compound lifts like squats, deadlifts, and chest presses, which spread the load across multiple large muscles. That way you're not overstressing any single muscle or joint. Safety is paramount here. Make sure you get expert instruction on load and technique. If you are new to lifting, book a few sessions with a trainer to learn proper technique and nail that down before adding weight.

LHS will not happen overnight. It can take months to build up to heavy loads if you are new. Expect to start with more moderate loads, lifting two to three sets of eight to fifteen reps to build a foundation and muscular endurance. After four to six weeks, you can bring the weight up and the repetitions down, so you're lifting five sets of five reps. When that becomes comfortable, you can aim for four to six sets of three to five reps.

OTHER TIPS FOR LIFTING HEAVY SH*T SUCCESSFULLY

WARM UP PROPERLY: You're going to be asking a lot of your muscles and joints, so make sure they are warmed up and ready for the job by easing into activity and gradually ramping up so your muscles are warmed up and primed for action. This is especially important during the menopausal years, when women have a higher incidence of joint pain due to increased inflammation and decreased muscle and connective tissue strength. Lifting will help (and not lifting makes it worse). You can also tamp down inflammation and pain with an anti-inflammatory diet (see chapter 10) and adaptogens (see chapter 4).

Your warm-up should include tissue care and mobility work like foam rolling and range-of-motion exercises. A good example of a 10- to 15-minute warm-up for a lifting session would be the following mobility session specially designed by Erin Carson.

As the strength trainer for endurance athletes like three-time Ironman World Champion Mirinda Carfrae, Erin's approach is to build her athletes up to be not just strong but energetic, nimble, and fast. She also practices what she preaches, recently running one of her fastest half-marathons at age 54. She's a co-owner and coach at RallySport in Boulder, Colorado, where she has worked for 27 years, and the head coach at ECFIT. So you know she knows her stuff!

FOAM ROLL LOWER LEG

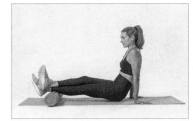 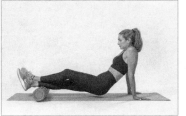

Sit on the floor with your legs straight out and crossed at the knee, hands on the floor behind you supporting your weight. Place the roller under the ankle of the lower leg. Slowly roll along the calf up and down from your ankle to your knee for 30 seconds. Then switch legs.

FOAM ROLL POSTERIOR HIP

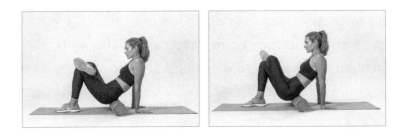

Sitting on the foam roller, cross your right ankle over your left knee and lean toward the right hip, putting your weight on your hands for support. Slowly roll your glutes back and forth over the roller for 30 seconds. Then switch sides.

OPEN HIP TOGGLE

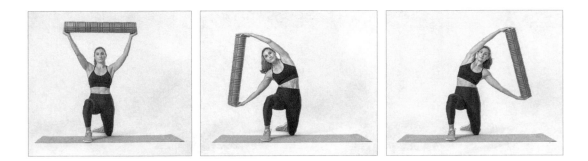

Kneel on a padded surface, holding a long foam roller overhead. Place your right leg in front of you so that your knees form 90-degree angles. Keeping your hips square, bend side to side from the waist, allowing your hips to sway gently. Repeat, alternating for 10 reps on each side. Then switch sides.

T SPINE EXTENSION

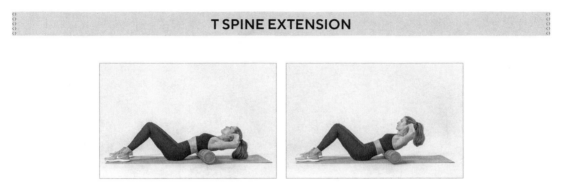

Lie back in an abdominal crunch position on the floor, knees bent, feet flat on the floor, arms bent, and hands behind your head, with your upper back draped over a long foam roller. Extend back and curl forward over the roller, massaging your upper back for 60 seconds.

DOWEL HIP OPENER

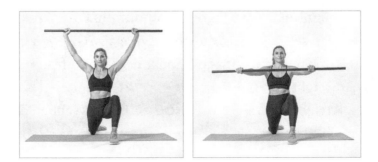

Kneel on a padded surface, holding a dowel overhead. Place your left leg in front of you so that your knees form 90-degree angles. Press your hips forward while reaching behind your head with the dowel. Then press your hips back while lowering the dowel in front of you. Repeat, alternating for 10 repetitions. Then switch sides.

TWIST HIP OPENER

Kneel on a padded surface, holding a light weight with both hands, arms stretched straight out from your chest. Place your right leg in front of you so that your knees form 90-degree angles. Simultaneously rotate toward the left while pressing your hips forward. Then return to start. Repeat for 10 reps. Then switch sides.

GIVE YOURSELF AMPLE REST BETWEEN SETS: LHS is not like circuit training, where you're jumping from move to move with minimal rest. You need *full, complete recovery* between sets to be ready to lift heavy again. Give yourself a minimum of two minutes if you're lifting six reps. You'll need up to five minutes for lower reps with heavier weight.

WEAVE LHS INTO YOUR OTHER WORKOUTS: Unless you're solely into power and strength sports like CrossFit, you're going to want to work your heavy lifting into your life in a way that allows you to feel strong and recovered for other activities like running, cycling, swimming, rock climbing, and so forth. Chapter 17 on exercise programming provides guidance on how to incorporate resistance training (as well as HIIT/SIT and plyometric training) into your existing training program for the best results.

CHECK WITH YOUR DOCTOR: If you've been diagnosed with osteoporosis or have bone or joint damage, consult with your medical professional first before lifting heavy weights. Though resistance training can help build bone, relieve arthritis pain, and make your skeleton and connective tissue stronger and more resilient, if you fall into a high-risk category, you might be better off sticking to the lower-rep range, especially if you're new to lifting. See chapter 16 for more on building bone if you have osteoporosis.

WHY AM I WETTING MYSELF?

Remember in chapter 3 when we talked about estrogen robbing connective tissue of elasticity and weakening the muscles of the pelvic floor? That's why you're more prone to leaking a little (or sometimes a lot) when you bear down to lift a heavy barbell off the floor or perform a fully weighted proper squat.

Kegel exercises are important. But they're just the beginning. The pelvic floor is an overlooked and underappreciated part of the core; it works in collaboration with the diaphragm, multifidus, and transversus abdominis (TrA) muscles, which form the shape of a canister. Ideally, all the muscles in this canister contract simultaneously to provide strength, support, and stability to your spine and organs whenever you move. Weak back or abdominal muscles, however, can contribute to incontinence, because the pelvic floor is forced to do more work than it was designed to handle.

That's why pelvic floor specialists like Chloë Murdock, a CSCS and physical therapist, make sure to improve the entire canister (the pelvic floor as well as the front, back, and sides of the core) to prevent this type of leaking.

A simple way to check if your TrA is working is to do a forearm plank, says Murdock. Can you keep your lower abdominal muscles flat? Or do they "dome" downwards?

"This doming is an indication that the TrA is not working well, and the superficial muscles are taking over instead," she says. Although classic planks are a good core-strengthening exercise, if you're doming, you should modify the exercise to make it easy enough that you can keep your lower abdomen flat. A simple fix is keeping your knees on the floor, or doing the plank at an incline with your arms on the edge of a couch.

Other "canister" strengthening exercises include:

KEGELS

These are the classic pelvic floor exercises. Clench your pelvic floor like you're trying to prevent yourself from wetting or soiling yourself. For the best results, you should include long, held squeezes as well as quick, short squeezes.

Aim to perform 10 long squeezes, holding each contraction for 10 seconds, followed by 10 short, strong squeezes. Like any muscle, your pelvic floor may not be strong enough to complete a full 20 reps. Do what you can today and work up to doing more as you go along. You can and should do pelvic floor work every day.

ELEVATOR ABS

Lie facedown with your arms bent out to the sides, hands folded under your forehead, palms down. Tighten your pelvic floor muscles, squeezing up as though trying to stop the flow of urine. Holding that contraction, tilt your pelvis and pull your diaphragm in as though trying to make it kiss your spine. Picture a string from the ceiling that is slowly lifting your back as you pull up and in as far as possible. Reverse the move, before finally releasing your pelvic floor muscles.

CHILD'S POSE BREATHING

The coordination of your diaphragm, abdominals, and pelvic floor is essential for bladder control and pressure management. You can work yours by performing deep breathing exercises in child's pose. Women who have done Kegels with no relief are often amazed at how quickly this strategy works. In fact, a study published in *Female Pelvic Medicine & Reconstructive Surgery* reported that women with incontinence issues who started practicing yoga moves targeted at pelvic floor health had a 71 percent decrease in total incontinence frequency after six weeks.

From a kneeling position, sit back on your heels and open your knees about hip-width. Bend forward, lowering your upper body between your thighs, allowing your forehead to rest on the floor. Extend your arms down along your calves, palms facing up. Breathe in deeply, expanding your rib cage, especially the lower rib cage, and exhale. Do 6 to 10 slow, even breaths.

For more on stopping the leaks, see chapter 17.

HEAVY LIFTING STAPLES

As mentioned previously, lifting heavy sh*t is done on big lifts, where you are spreading out the load over multiple muscle groups. Here are some LHS staples to work into your routine.

SQUAT

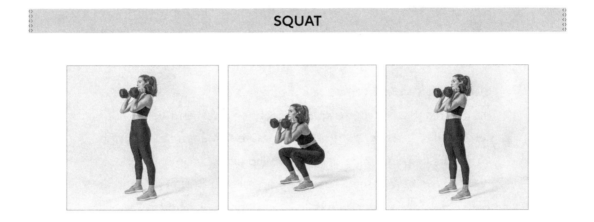

You can start using dumbbells, as shown. As you master the move, advance to a barbell squat for the full effect. One study found that cyclists who added heavy squatting exercises to their regular training routine improved their cycling time-to-exhaustion at maximum aerobic power by 17.2 percent after just eight weeks.

DO IT: Stand with your feet hip- to shoulder-width apart, with your toes pointed slightly out. Hold weights at your shoulders or down at your sides. Push your butt and hips back as if you were sitting in a chair and lower down as far as possible while keeping your weight on your heels. Return to the starting position and repeat.

Though you can do this move with dumbbells, for the full-body effect try it with a barbell (after mastering proper technique). When using a barbell, the bar should sit across the back of your shoulders, resting on your trap muscles, with your hands gripping the bar on either side of your shoulders.

Other squat variations to try:

SPLIT SQUAT

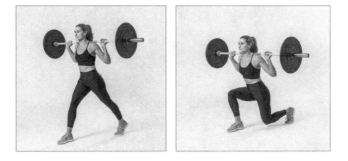

Holding weight at your sides (if dumbbells) or across your back (if a barbell), stand tall and take a giant step forward with one foot, planting the forward foot so that both heels are firmly on the ground, toes pointed forward. Maintain an upright torso as you bend both your knees, allowing the back heel to lift off the ground as you lower your body until your back shin and front thigh are parallel to the ground. Return to start. Complete a set, then switch sides.

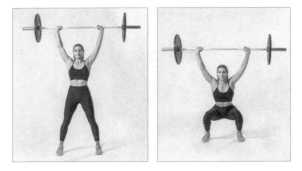

This is an advanced move. It demands a strong core and good stability (and also helps develop both). It's best to start with an unloaded barbell or even a dowel when you're first getting started. Position yourself as you would for a back squat, but with your hands slightly wider, so they are closer to the outside of the bar where the plates are. Bend your knees and drop your hips just enough to engage your lower body muscles and then powerfully extend your knees and hips and drive the barbell overhead, fully extending your arms in a Y. Keeping your core tight and chest up, press your hips back and start squatting down as far as possible while maintaining form. Return to start.

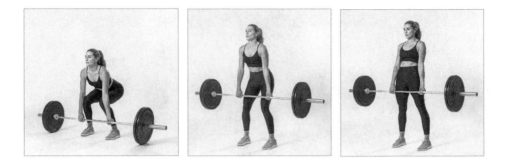

Deadlifting builds strong glutes, which are the lifeblood of endurance athletes, though too often it's also their weak link. Exercise studies find that deadlifts beat planks when it comes to developing your deep abdominal muscles that give you rock-solid core strength—something every athlete can use.

DO IT: Place a barbell on the floor in front of you. Stand with feet hip-width apart, toes pointing forward. Keeping your back flat, hinge at the hips and lower toward the floor, allowing your knees to bend naturally to grasp the barbell, so your arms are on either side of your legs. Press into the floor and lift the weight off the floor, keeping the weight close to your body, contracting your glutes, and pushing your hips forward to a standing position. Keep the weight close to your body and lower it back to the floor until your upper body is almost parallel to the floor. Repeat.

Other deadlift variations to try:

SUMO DEADLIFT

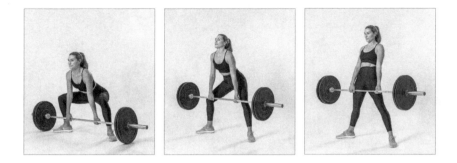

As the name implies, sumo deadlifts are done with a wider stance than the traditional deadlift. You start by assuming a wide stance with your toes slightly pointed out. Then hinge at the hips as you would for a traditional deadlift, only this time keep your arms inside of your legs. Perform a deadlift as you normally would. Sumo deadlifts are easier on the lower back and, according to a 2019 study published in the *Journal of Sports Science and Medicine,* may be a better option for less experienced deadlifters who have longer torsos.

SINGLE LEG DEADLIFT

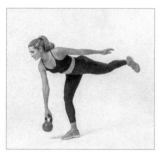

This deadlift variation improves balance and stability while strengthening your back, core, and legs. Stand tall, holding a weight in your right hand down at your side, with your left hand on your hip or by your side. Shift your weight to your right leg, allowing the leg to have a natural soft bend in the knee, and press your left leg back while simultaneously hinging at the waist and tipping your torso forward and dropping the weight toward the floor until your upper body is nearly parallel to the floor. Your body should form a straight line from your head to your heel. Then draw the left leg forward and lift your torso back to the starting position. Complete a set and switch legs.

BENCH PRESS

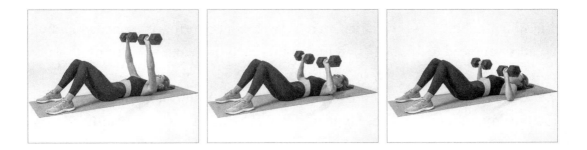

Too many women neglect their upper body in their resistance training routines. To maintain strength, build bone density, and have support for your primary activities, whether they're endurance- or power-based, you need to lift heavy sh*t with your upper body too. The bench press is a classic strength training exercise for strengthening your chest, shoulders, and triceps.

DO IT: You can start using dumbbells on a bench or the floor, as shown. As you master the move, advance to a barbell press. To do it, lie flat on your back on a bench. Grip the bar with your hands wider than shoulder-width apart. Lift the bar off the rack and lower it slowly down to your mid-chest. Push through your chest and push the weight toward the ceiling so that your arms are fully extended. Repeat.

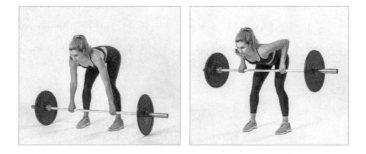

This move strengthens your upper and mid-back muscles. So it's good for posture and spinal stability. This variation on the classic bent-over row is more demanding because you need to lift the bar off the ground each time, and you also need to use proper form, rather than rely on momentum, for each rep.

DO IT: Bend forward, hinging at the hips, until your back is parallel to the ground. Your knees should be slightly bent. Grasp the bar using an overhand grip, with your hands just wider than shoulder-width apart. Brace your core and squeeze your shoulder blades as you lift the weight up to your torso. Then lower the bar all the way back to the floor, making sure that your back stays parallel to the floor throughout the move.

WHERE DOES CROSSFIT FIT IN?

Looking at a schedule that includes LHS, HIIT, and plyometrics, CrossFit athletes always ask: "Where does CrossFit fit in?" After all, anyone who does CrossFit knows that any given workout can include all three! The real trick when you're including CrossFit in your schedule is to *not* do the same types of workouts day in and day out. This is where women (and men!) can reach a point where they're just always tired and not making progress because they can't really nail the hard workouts like they should and they're not allowing themselves any recovery.

You can choose to do the MetCon (metabolic conditioning) elements of CrossFit as your HIIT workouts and the lifting elements of the class as your LHS. But it's best to only focus on one per class. If your focus for the day is LHS, prioritize that element of the class and go super, super easy on the MetCon portion, just flushing out your system. On days that you are focusing on HIIT, go all in on the MetCon, but use the lifting portion of the class only to work on technique.

LIFT YEAR-ROUND

At this point in life, you need to strength-train year-round, not just in the off-season or during the winter months or whenever you're not participating in your primary activities such as running, cycling, swimming, or other sports.

Ideally, you should be lifting two to three days a week. If you're an endurance athlete, you can lift twice a week in season by combining your LHS sessions with your SIT interval work. Do your lifting first to potentiate all your muscles. That way, when you hit the intervals, you're able to get high intensity under load to promote better adaptations for racing.

Unless strength training is your primary activity, you want to use LHS to complement your primary sport, not to replace or detract from it. That means scheduling yourself so that your hardest lifting days are separate from your long endurance days to give yourself ample recovery time.

BRACE YOURSELF

A properly braced neutral spine is the bedrock from which all safe, dynamic, and high-volume athletic movement is generated, says Dr. Kelly Starrett, a coach, physiotherapist, and author of *Becoming a Supple Leopard*. He teaches the following bracing sequence, which was originally published in *ROAR*. I highly recommend that all women practice until it becomes automatic; it's especially important as a complement to LHS because maintaining proper form and posture is paramount to performing the moves safely. The beauty of this sequence is that it starts with your feet and works systematically up to your head to ensure that you address any improper postures that you might have adopted over time. Practice this sequence on its own a few times a day and employ it before strength training.

STEP 1: SCREW YOUR FEET INTO THE GROUND
Position your feet directly under your hips and parallel to each other. Now screw your feet into the ground by exerting force in an outward direction from your hips. Externally rotate your right hip and press your right foot into the ground in a clockwise direction and externally rotate your left hip and press your left foot into the ground in a counterclockwise position.

STEP 2: SQUEEZE YOUR BUTT

Set your pelvis in the proper, neutral position by squeezing your glutes. Activate your glutes and then reduce the tension to maintain a neutral pelvic position.

STEP 3: INHALE AND LOCK IT IN

Your glutes set your pelvis in position and your abs lock it in. Lock your pelvis and rib cage in place by taking a big breath in through your diaphragm with your glutes squeezed.

STEP 4: EXHALE AND BALANCE YOUR RIB CAGE

As you exhale, balance your rib cage over your pelvis and tighten your belly. You're not sucking in or drawing in your belly. You're stiffening it into place as you exhale. This creates intra-abdominal pressure around your spine.

STEP 5: NEUTRALIZE YOUR HEAD AND SHOULDERS

Rotate your shoulders back, widen your collarbones, and turn your palms up toward the sky. As you do, center your head over your shoulders, focusing your eyes forward. The goal is to set your head and shoulders in a neutral position and align your ears over your shoulders, hips, and ankles.

STEP 6: STAND FULLY BRACED

Let your arms fall to your sides so that your thumbs point forward and your shoulders remain externally rotated. You should be standing with your ears over your shoulders, your rib cage over your pelvis, and your hips over your knees and ankles, fully braced and ready to go.

NEXT LEVEL MENOPAUSE MAKEOVER:
COMING BACK FROM MEDICALLY INDUCED MENOPAUSE

CHERYL,* 38, is a competitive cyclist and CrossFit enthusiast, but after being through medically induced menopause, she doesn't feel like much of either. Her goal is to get her strength and energy levels back where they used to be.

GENERAL ASSESSMENT

Cheryl was diagnosed with breast cancer when she was 35. Now, at age 38, 18 months post chemotherapy and in a state of medically induced menopause, she finds herself in a body she barely recognizes. She's 5'8" and 141 pounds, which is normal for her height. But she went from a body fat of 15 percent to 26 percent, and her power is down dramatically. She is still on Tamoxifen, but otherwise, she is through with her treatments and eager to improve her body composition, regain her strength, and restore her energy levels.

She works from home, so she has a lot of freedom to schedule her meals. But she's definitely a little lost and doesn't have a grasp on how to fuel around training and for building lean mass. Her fitness and exercise tolerance are still pretty low, but she tries to lift or ride every day. She is very consistent and disciplined about scheduling herself, but now she needs more specificity instead of the general sessions she does day in and day out. She wants to lean more heavily into the competitive cycling scene, so we decide to first increase her overall strength with heavy lifting (rather than all the CrossFit) and work on aerobic capacity, and also stimulate lean mass development. Then we'll shift her work toward building cycling-specific fitness.

We also wanted to establish some good fueling and nutrition habits, especially surrounding her training. We'll increase her protein and adjust carbohydrates. Since she is more insulin resistant following the medically induced menopause, we shift the carbohydrates toward nutrient-dense, fiber-rich sources, like seasonal fruits and veggies and oats and other whole grains, on long aerobic training days.

Finally, her gut had taken a beating during chemotherapy and cancer treatment. So we want to make sure everything she is eating is going to be beneficial for rebuilding a diverse, healthy gut microbiome. We include some fermented foods like kefir or kombucha every day.

HER NEW ROUTINE

Here's how her new schedule looks after our makeover:

MONDAY: 7:30 to 11:30 a.m. work. Instead of CrossFit, she goes to the gym and does a heavy lifting session including squats, deadlifts, and core work. She rides her bike to and from the gym, which gives her a little spin out to flush her muscles after the session.

TUESDAY: Instead of the long, easy ride, she does a hard gym day of CrossFit followed immediately by a SIT session on the Assault Bike: 5-minute warm-up / 3 rounds of 8 x 30 seconds (100 percent functional threshold power, or FTP) / 15 seconds (50 percent FTP). Repeat 8 times.

WEDNESDAY: 7:30 to 11:30 a.m. work. Super easy training day, including a 60 minute mellow lunch spin and 30 minutes of restorative yoga in the evening.

THURSDAY: Moderately hard morning training day. CrossFit at lunch followed by Assault Bike intervals: 3 minutes on / 90 seconds off; 2 minutes on / 1 minute off; 1 minute on / 30 seconds off and a 3 to 5 minute spin between sets. (Or she can do a hill repeat session instead of the assault bike intervals). Then off to work from noon to whenever.

FRIDAY: 7:30 to 11:30 a.m. work. Moderately hard training day. Instead of CrossFit, she does an easy 30 to 45 minute spin, followed by 4 rounds of 10 box jumps, 10 kettlebell swings, and 10/10 kettlebell alternating leg.

SATURDAY: Easy 2 hour endurance ride or day off.

SUNDAY: Day off (or 2 hour easy endurance ride if she took Saturday off).

THE RESULTS

After four months, Cheryl's doing much better. She has dropped a little weight, down to 137 from 141, but more importantly, she has really improved her body composition, down to 18 percent from 26 percent fat. She's built back some of her lean mass while losing some body fat.

She's feeling strong in the gym and she's back on the bike, slowly building back her aerobic base and endurance. Cheryl feels in control and on the right track again.

7

GET A JUMP ON MENOPAUSAL STRENGTH LOSSES

How to (literally) bound into a powerful future.

Society has traditionally perceived aging women as frail "little old ladies" who need assistance opening doors and carrying groceries. We get the message loud and clear that as we get older, we need to take it easy and be careful because we might get hurt or break ourselves.

So I ask, is it any wonder that, when treated this way, we so often expect to turn into frail women who need assistance? Can you say self-fulfilling prophecy? It's because of this deeply ingrained messaging that women often look aghast when they see that I have put plyometric training (also known as jump training) front and center in my "Menopause for Athletes" programming. We've been taught that we should be taking it down a notch, not turning it up. But that is just not true.

In fact, a 2019 systematic research review of the recent literature on plyometrics and older adults ranging in age from 58 to 79 reported that plyometrics often improved muscular strength, bone health, body composition, posture, and physical performance. None of the studies reported increased injuries or other adverse events from plyometric exercises among participants. The researchers concluded, "Plyometric training is a feasible and safe training option with potential for improving various performance, functional, and health-related outcomes in older persons."

To be clear: plyometrics is not all about jumping on and off high boxes (though if you're already doing that, I won't tell you to stop!). It's about impact. It's about jumping, hopping, bounding, or otherwise purposefully giving your bones and muscles the extra stimulus that comes when you push off against gravity and land back down. It is those impacts—big or small—that generate positive results.

Let me also be clear that, unless you've already been engaged in some form of jump training, I'm not going to recommend that you start doing lots of bounding or jumping right out of the gate. You need to build up to it. But you absolutely should lay the groundwork and start building up to including plyometrics as a regular part of your training regime because it will help you maintain and improve your sports performance as well as your general well-being. And no, running is not enough. We are talking about multi-directional force and impact to garner the benefits that jump-training has to offer.

SWITCH ON YOUR FAST AND STRONG GENES

As you've already learned, estrogen is anabolic and helps you create forceful muscle contractions. It helps you generate power. As we lose estrogen, our muscles get smaller and weaker. A 2018 Finnish study of more than 900 women found that menopausal status is significantly associated with reduced muscle strength and vertical jump height.

Without estrogen, your body needs a strong stimulus to pick up the slack and keep your muscle fibers strong and firing quickly and powerfully. That's where plyometrics comes in. The reason plyometrics works so well is that it triggers what are known as epigenetic changes. Without jumping too far into the scientific deep end (pun intended), when you are exposed to any kind of stress, your body experiences some changes in your genes. Certain genes start switching on or off. Sometimes those changes are harmful, as with cigarette smoking, and sometimes they're helpful, as with exercise.

When you do plyometrics, you wake up some otherwise very quiet genes inside your muscle cells that stimulate those cells to improve power and even the composition of the muscle itself in a way that improves the integrity of the muscle, its contractile strength, and its response and reaction time.

This is extremely important because we lose our speed and power—the strong fast-twitch muscle contraction—not only with age but specifically at the onset of menopause. We want to do what we can to maintain our speed, our ability to sprint, and our ability to bound up stairs.

BUILD MITOCHONDRIA POWER

Plyometrics also maintains, builds, and improves the function of your mitochondria—those energy-producing powerhouses in your cells. When you have more mitochondria and better mitochondrial function, you have more fuel available to keep producing energy and power. That makes you a better endurance athlete and also preserves metabolic health.

Speaking of metabolic health, plyometrics improves insulin sensitivity, so you can get glucose into your cells, where you need it, instead of keeping it in your fat stores, where you don't. The fast velocity and energetics of plyometrics instigates more of the glucose transporter type 4 (GLUT4) transporters to be activated on the plasma membrane of muscle and fat cells. This way, you rely less on insulin to get the glucose where it needs to be. That improves your exercise performance and body composition and helps prevent chronic conditions like heart disease and diabetes.

CREATE A STRONG SKELETON

As you know, estrogen plays an important role in bone development and maintenance. Research shows that women can lose up to 20 percent of their bone density within the first five to seven years postmenopause as estrogen levels decline. That's one-fifth of your skeletal strength. Resistance training helps. But to really improve bone, you need to jump.

In a 2015 study of 60 women published in the *American Journal of Health Promotion*, researchers found that jumping just 10 to 20 times a day significantly improved bone density in the hips after 16 weeks. The women who jumped 20 times twice a day had greater improvements in bone mineral density than those doing 10 jumps twice a day, but both groups fared better than the non jumpers who lost bone mineral density over the course of the study.

While running helps build bones, it's far less effective than jumping, according to research. That's because running creates mostly one-directional stress as you're moving forward in the same place. It's too similar to the stress that your bones get when you walk and perform most daily tasks. Remember, your body adapts to the type of stress you generally put on it. So if you want your bones to adapt to be stronger, they need novel stimulus too. Research has confirmed that postmenopausal women should be encouraged to do jumping exercises to build bone density.

So unless you play tennis, squash, or basketball (in which case you're already doing a lot of multidirectional jumping), you don't have enough stress hitting your bones at every angle to promote bone growth. Jumping in different directions, on the other hand, creates a stronger impact and sends signals to the bones that they need to remodel to get stronger to handle the stress. This is particularly important for cyclists, swimmers, and women who do mostly non-impact sports that put no impact stress on the skeleton.

Though jump training has been shown to be safe and effective for people with low bone density, if you've already been diagnosed with osteoporosis, you may need to consult with your doctor regarding plyometrics.

For more on building strong bones, see chapter 16.

JUMP TO IT

Like all strong medicine, you only need a small amount of plyometrics to reap the benefits. Just 10 minutes three times a week is all the jumping you need. I like to just finish off my strength training with a short plyometric circuit. As a bonus, I feel energized for the day.

It's important to phase in jump training according to your ability. You want to be sure that your connective tissues are conditioned and ready for the impact, so start slow and easy.

The simplest move to start with is:

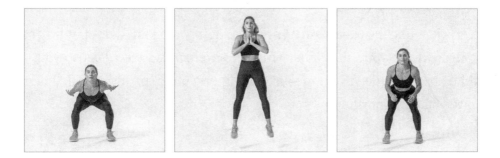

Stand with your feet wider than shoulder-width, feet turned out a little. Extend your arms straight in front of you. Squat down, extending your arms behind you, until your butt drops below knee level. Quickly extend your legs and jump into the air. Land softly, immediately dropping into another squat. Repeat 8 to 10 times. Start with one set. Work up to two. You can do one set in the morning and one in the evening. All that matters is you get in your jumping.

Once you're comfortable with the squat jump, you can move to circuit training: performing a number of jump exercises one after the next. A sample circuit would be 45 seconds "on" (jumping) and 15 seconds "off" (resting between jumps), aiming for three circuits with five minutes' rest between them. If you're just starting out, do one circuit and gradually work your way up over the course of a few weeks. If you're more advanced, you can aim for two or three circuits.

JUMPING JACKS

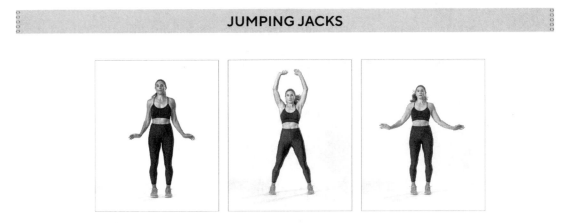

Yep, this is just like the classic you remember doing as a kid! Start standing straight with your arms by your side. Then jump up and spread your legs so you land in a straddle stance while simultaneously bringing your arms overhead. Then jump back to the starting position.

SIDE HOPS

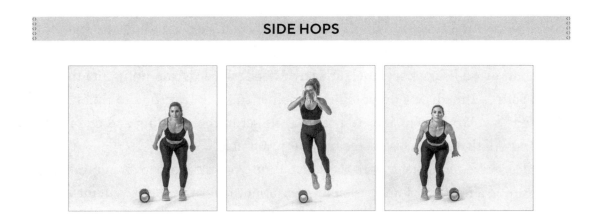

Place a rolled-up towel or other object (just be sure you can clear it) on the floor and stand next to it. Bend your knees, swing your arms back and jump up and sideways over the towel, swinging your arms up to chest level as you do. Land softly and immediately bend at the knees and jump right back to the starting position. Repeat.

SKIPPING

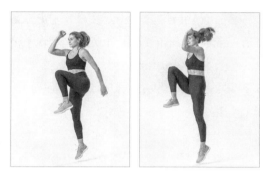

Skip just as you did when you were a kid, but use your arms to propel yourself upward and drive your bent knee forward and up to get as much height as possible on each skip. This is best done on a soft surface, not concrete. You can do this in place as a single leg hop if you don't have room (or don't want to skip down the block).

Start with your feet hip-distance apart. Drive your left knee upward, propelling off the floor and gaining as much height as possible, while swinging your right arm overhead. Land softly and immediately switch legs and arms. Alternate throughout the set.

Next you can move to an intermediate circuit:

SWITCH LEG LUNGES

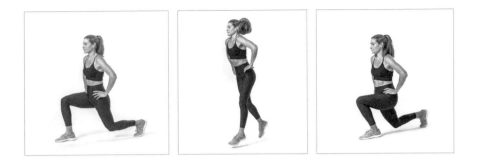

Lunge forward to where your right thigh is parallel to the floor. With hands on your hips or swinging your arms for balance and momentum, jump up and switch legs, landing in a lunge with your left foot forward.

If you have a history of knee problems, do a shallower lunge, where you don't bend your knees a full 90 degrees.

MOUNTAIN CLIMBER

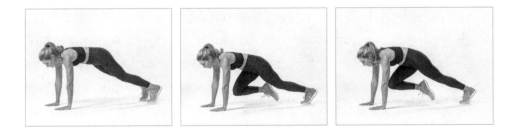

Start in a high plank, arms and legs extended, hands on the floor shoulder-width apart, with your body forming a straight line from your head to your heels. Keeping your core tight, drive your left knee in toward your chest. Extend your left leg back to starting position while simultaneously driving your right knee toward your chest. Continue switching legs, so that it feels like you're horizontally running in place.

SUMO SQUAT JUMPS

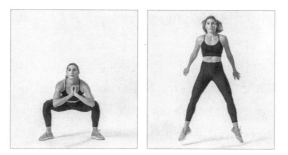

Stand with your legs in a wide stance, feet turned out at 45 degrees. Bend your knees into a plié, then jump up explosively, keeping your core engaged. Land with soft knees, lowering your body back into the sumo squat position and immediately jump again.

Once you get comfortable with the intermediate circuit, you can proceed to a more advanced circuit:

TUCK JUMP

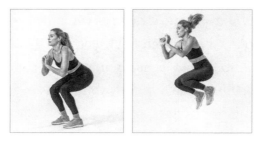

Similar to a squat jump, the tuck jump uses your arms to explode up and bring your knees in as high and as close to your body as you can.

Stand with your feet wider than shoulder-width, feet turned out a little. Squat down until your butt drops below knee level. Quickly extend your legs and jump into the air, bringing your knees up toward your chest. Land softly, immediately dropping into another squat.

If that is too intense, you can start with Burpees. Begin in a squat position with your hands on the floor in front of you. Kick your feet back into a push-up position. Immediately return your feet to the squat position. Leap as high as possible from the squat position. Land softly, keeping your feet, knees, and hips in alignment and feet pointed straight ahead. Repeat.

SPEED SKATER

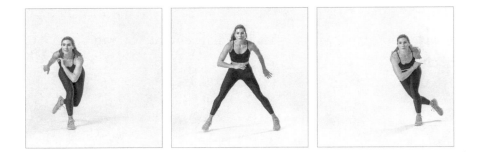

Stand with your feet shoulder-width apart, knees slightly bent. Shift your weight onto your right leg, bending it about 45 degrees while sweeping your left leg behind you. In one smooth motion, sweep your left leg back to the left and jump from your right leg to your left, immediately bending into a half squat with your left leg as you sweep your right behind you. Crisscross your arms in front of your body like a speed skater as you jump from side to side.

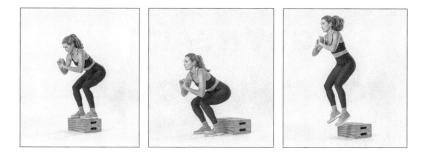

Stand on a step or small box. Using your arms for power, jump off the step and land with your knees slightly bent and feet hip-width apart. Immediately jump explosively up into the air (*not* back onto the step). Step back onto the step and repeat. This is the opposite of a box jump, which is an advanced move. Once you get super-comfortable with plyometrics you can try box jumping:

Stand facing a 12- to 18-inch-high box or step. Squat down and jump up using a double arm swing to propel your body. Land firmly on the box, with knees soft to absorb the impact. Step down and repeat.

AQUA JUMPING FOR BAD JOINTS

Can't do plyometric exercises because of an existing injury? It's beyond the scope of this book to advise the appropriate course of action for every individual, but you can get the motions down by doing your plyo exercises in the shallow end of the swimming pool as a form of HIIT. Work with your physical therapist on the best way to work up to some impact.

8

GUT HEALTH
FOR ATHLETIC GLORY

*Nutrition for health and performance
starts with digestion.*

Selene's Nana, standing over the stove for much of the day, would regale her with the old saying: "The way to a man's heart is through his stomach." Today we have moved on from many of the underlying implications of that classic piece of grandmotherly wisdom, but there's actually some real science to be found in it. Both physically and emotionally, the way to anyone's heart (including your own!) is through the stomach. And for menopausal women, it's also the way to improve mood, energy balance, sleep, body composition, immunity, health, and athletic performance.

Whatever your goal, achieving it starts with your gut—or more specifically, your gut microbiome. Research on the gut microbiome has exploded over the past five to ten years. Not only is your gut microbiome essential for basic digestion and GI health, but the garden in your gut influences your entire being. Instead of wondering, *What am I going to eat to be healthy?* your first thought should actually be, *How is the food I am choosing going to affect my gut microbiome?* Because it all starts there.

THE GUT MICROBIOME BASICS

Your gut microbiome is the universe of microorganisms that live in your intestinal tract. The medical community once thought that these little microbes were important primarily for good digestion and nutrient absorption. They understood that you didn't want them escaping from the intestines (such as you see with "leaky gut syndrome" when intestinal inflammation increases intestinal permeability), because that could lead to a bad infection or even sepsis of the blood. But now we know that there's a direct link between what is happening in your gut and what is happening throughout your body, including your brain.

When you eat, you feed your microbiome before you feed yourself because those microbes assist in breaking down and absorbing food. As part of this process, they also generate important by-products that help you produce hormones and regulate your metabolism as well as your central nervous system and automatic nervous system function.

When you have a diverse, balanced microbiome, you have good health and performance. When your gut microbiome gets out of balance, you end up with a greater risk for obesity, metabolic and cardiovascular disease, anxiety, depression, and other diseases. About 60 percent of your immunity originates in your gut. It literally affects everything.

Take sleep as an example. You probably would never imagine that the flora in your intestines would affect your sleep. But if you have an overabundance of microbiome bacteria that stimulate your sympathetic nervous system, you will be unable to fall into that short-wave reparative sleep; you'll end up with less REM sleep, spending more time in light sleep, and your health, recovery, and performance will suffer. Given that menopause already disrupts sleep, you can see how important it is to protect your sleep through every other possible avenue—including the gut microbiome.

Another unexpected benefit of a healthy microbiome is brain health. Some of the by-products of a healthy gut microbiome help stimulate the production of brain-derived neurotrophic factor (BDNF), which, as mentioned in chapters 3 and 5, helps build brain cells and preserves healthy cognition. This gut-brain axis is proving more important than we'd ever imagined. This is especially true for menopausal women, since declining hormones can cause the mental slump we call brain fog.

When it comes to your performance, research shows that a healthy gut microbiome can improve your metabolism, energy availability during exercise, and recovery after a workout.

12 KEY BENEFITS OF A HEALTHY GUT MICROBIOME

There are myriad benefits of a healthy gut microbiome. For menopausal women, a healthy gut microbiome offsets the detrimental effects of hormone fluctuation and decline, while improving performance and health on so many levels, including:

- Mental strength
- Body composition
- Bone density and remodeling
- Ability to absorb and use nutrients
- Sleep quality, especially REM and restorative sleep
- Natural antioxidant production
- Ability to build mitochondria

- Energy management and metabolism and reduced fatigue
- Reduced inflammation
- Improved energy
- Improved lactic acid breakdown (enabling you to exercise harder and longer)
- Increased ATP levels for quick, powerful energy production

GUT MICROBIOME BALANCE AND BODY COMPOSITION

Among the women who come to me, the most common complaint about menopause has to do with body composition. Even if they don't have hot flashes or night sweats, they often notice an unfavorable shift in muscle and fat. As research on the gut microbiome evolves, it appears that the ratio of bacteria you have in your gut has a profound impact on your body composition.

Ninety percent of your gut microbiota are two types: Firmicutes and Bacteroidetes. These two families of microbiota have a pronounced impact on your weight and your health.

Specifically, Firmicutes are sugar junkies. They want nothing more than to sit down in front of some Saturday morning cartoons with a bowl of chocolate-coated sugar pops, and they'll send signals to your brain to keep the sugary snacks coming. Eventually the abundance of sugar is converted to fat. Firmicutes also generate inflammation in the body and can slow down metabolism. Evolutionarily speaking, these bacteria probably served us well during times of famine, when we'd consume high amounts of high-sugar foods when we found them, creating fat stores to carry us through to our next feeding. Firmicutes are far less useful today. In fact, research finds that a higher ratio of Firmicutes within the gastrointestinal tract is linked to obesity. On the other side, Bacteroidetes block inflammation and raise your metabolism. People who have more Bacteroidetes within their gut flora are less likely to be obese.

These bacteria also regulate how much energy we absorb from the food we eat and deposit into our fat cells. Firmicutes absorb more, and Bacteroidetes absorb less. So if you have a higher proportion of Firmicutes in your gut, you will be more apt to gain weight than someone with a higher portion of Bacteroidetes, even if you eat the exact same diet.

That's right: body composition is far more complex than the oversimplified "calories in, calories out" dictum we've been led to believe. Research shows that Firmicutes-dominant gut microbiomes are associated with obesity and related diseases. Firmicutes may also increase inflammation, which contributes to weight gain and chronic disease. Having a Bacteroidetes-dominant gut, on the other hand, is associated with having a leaner body composition.

The difference can be pronounced. In one instance, a woman gained 34 pounds in 16 months and went from being normal weight (BMI 26.4) to obese (BMI 33) after receiving a fecal transplant that unfavorably changed her microbiome.

Studies show that calorie restriction and fasting in the non-active population may shift microbiota composition to a more favorable Bacteroidetes-to-Firmicutes ratio. But we are talking here about active women. The best way for active women to build a healthy, diverse, balanced microbiome is through microbiome-building foods and exercise habits, and also by paying close attention to the food they eat before, during, and after exercise.

FEEDING YOUR MICROBIOME

First and foremost, you need a whole-food diet with plenty of plants for your bacteria to eat. Eating plenty of fibrous fruits and vegetables increases the diversity of your microbiome. A large-scale international 2021 study from King's College in London confirmed that eating a diet rich in plant-based foods encourages the presence of gut microbes that are linked to a lower risk of heart disease and other common illnesses.

A big plus for menopausal women is that these foods also increase the bacteria that use estrone (the less desirable form of estrogen) as a primary fuel source. Two trickle-down benefits of this are fewer menopausal symptoms and a decreased risk of cancer. For optimum health and menopausal benefits, you should be aiming for at least 25 grams of fiber from plant foods every day.

Foods that are rich in micronutrients known as polyphenols are also excellent for creating a healthy Bacteroidetes-to-Firmicutes balance. Some of the top foods with polyphenols are fruits (especially berries), vegetables, nuts, seeds, beans, dark chocolate, coffee, tea, olive oil, and red wine. Research on more than 1,400 men and women presented at United European Gastroenterology Week 2019 showed that eating a diet rich in plant-based foods, such as the ones just mentioned, and also including grains, legumes, and fish was linked to a healthier gut microbiota as well as lower levels of inflammation. Taking all this into consideration, it's not surprising that eating a Mediterranean-style diet (which is brimming with fruits, veggies, and whole foods) is good for your gut.

Also, there's good news for coffee lovers: coffee consumption is linked to a healthier gut microbiome, according to other research presented at the American College of Gastroenterology annual meeting in 2019. This study, which actually took gut microbiome samples directly from various parts of the colon during colonoscopies (most studies examine stool samples), found that people who drink two or more cups of coffee a day have a healthier gut microbiome than those who drink less or no coffee. The microbiomes of coffee drinkers had a greater abundance of bacterial species that are richer in anti-inflammatory properties and were considerably less likely to harbor the bacteria that have been linked to obesity and other metabolic conditions. These gut microbiome benefits may be one of the myriad reasons that coffee consumption is linked to a lower risk of dying from all causes.

Of course, we can't talk about gut health without mentioning probiotics, which are foods that contain healthy bacteria. You can maintain your gut microbiome diversity by eating a wide variety of probiotic foods, which contain healthy bacteria that can colonize your gut in a positive way, such as fermented foods like yogurt, kefir, sauerkraut, kombucha, and tempeh. Note, however, that even though yogurt naturally contains certain probiotics, some manufacturers add more probiotics, especially Lactobacillus acidophilus. Avoid yogurts with these added probiotics. Eating more of any one strain than you need can cause an imbalance, which is counterproductive to gut health.

Probiotics go hand in hand with prebiotics, which are the foods that are particularly good at keeping those probiotic bacteria thriving. Excellent prebiotic sources include garlic, onions, leeks, asparagus, green bananas, dandelion greens, and Jerusalem artichoke.

What you don't need are probiotic or prebiotic supplements. Though probiotic supplements have a large number of bacteria, they are often not diverse, and you may not need the bacteria you're taking in supplemental form. We also don't know the long-term effects of taking these supplements, which could trigger a backlash similar to what happens with antibiotics and throw your microbiome out of balance. The only time you may benefit from taking supplements is after taking antibiotics or other medications that have wiped out your gut flora and you need to build it back up. The same goes for prebiotic supplements. These products are expensive, and you may not need to promote the growth of the bacteria that they are designed to feed.

Finally, go easy on processed food and refined carbohydrates. Research has shown that people whose diets are rich in processed fast food and refined sugar have fewer good types of bacteria in their guts, as well as more intestinal inflammation.

EXERCISING YOUR MICROBIOME

Regular exercise promotes a diverse, healthy gut microbiome. When you're working out, you reduce the amount of oxygen and increase the heat in your gut. This environment allows some bacteria to grow and stunts the growth of others. Specifically, Bacteroidetes tend to rise and Firmicutes tend to be shut down. To increase lean mass and decrease excess body fat, that's what you want. But if you are feeding your gut simple sugars like sugary sports drinks, chews, gels, blocks, and candies during exercise, you're feeding Firmicutes, which can promote the overgrowth of these bad boys.

When you're done exercising, the communication between your gut and your brain along the gut-brain axis also boosts the bacteria that improve your GI lining so that it can block the wrong type of bacteria from getting into your gut and keep the right bacteria in.

Research published in the journal *Gut* reported that athletes have a higher diversity of gut microorganisms than their sedentary peers. Their microbiome is also healthier. In fact, in one study, just six weeks of exercising 30 to 60 minutes three times a week significantly reduced the number of inflammation-causing microbes and increased the beneficial microbes in a group of previously sedentary (but not overweight) volunteers.

In what could be considered a positive feedback loop, the beneficial changes in your gut microbiome from exercise also improve your exercise performance. Research on Boston marathon runners found that, compared to nonrunners, their guts had a higher population of bacteria from the genus Veillonella. Veillonella bacteria eat lactate as their main dietary staple. That's particularly helpful for exercise because, when lactate accumulates, our muscles become fatigued.

But there's a tipping point, and what you eat during exercise, especially once you start crossing the line from moderate to longer endurance exercise bouts, is important to maintaining that healthy diversity and balance.

Extreme exercise, like ultras and Ironman, increases inflammation above and beyond typical, healthy levels that the body can adapt to. It can lead to an abundance of bacteria that thrive in this unbalanced environment and perpetuate that inflammation. If you're not careful with what you eat and don't give yourself adequate recovery after intense exercise, you can really wreck your gut.

Specifically, foods common to sports nutrition can play havoc with your gut microbiome. As mentioned earlier, simple carbs and highly processed energy foods feed Firmicutes. Before you know it, your GI tract is inflamed and your microbiome is seriously out of balance as the increase in Firmicutes triggers more sugar cravings to feed them. That sets you up for decreased energy, slower recovery, mood swings, and more muscle soreness. Pretty much the opposite of what you want!

This is why understanding the mechanics of sports nutrition is super-important. Knowing that you're at a higher risk for throwing your gut microbiome out of whack, you want to think carefully about what you are eating before and after training and about the foods you use to fuel those long days of moderate to high activity. You want to save the super-processed carbs and simple sugars for when you really need a quick hit of energy, like toward the end of a race. Otherwise, you need to be consuming real food that contains a mix of macronutrients. In the following chapters, we'll dive deeper into what to eat and when.

NEXT LEVEL MENOPAUSE MAKEOVER:
A BUSY DOCTOR GETS HER BODY BACK

JUDY,* 48, came to me with one goal: get fit, so she could feel better and be the role model to her patients that she wanted to be.

GENERAL ASSESSMENT

At 5'9," 161 pounds, and between 25 to 28 percent body fat (depending on the time of year and where she was in her training), Judy was already in a generally healthy range. But her menopausal symptoms were definitely getting in her way and shifting her body composition in a negative direction for her. Despite her regular exercise regime, she wasn't seeing any improvement in her strength, body composition, or energy levels.

She was 47 at the time and had been experiencing disruptive symptoms for about a year at that point. She'd had a marked increase in belly and breast fat, and the quality of her sleep had deteriorated significantly. Even though she has a high-stress job, she used to be able to fall asleep and stay asleep. Now, she was waking up all the time. She was having hot flashes, especially in the evening and in the middle of the night (further disrupting her sleep). She was also suffering from brain fog that was interfering with her clinical work—she would be assessing her patients and suddenly not able to find basic words and terms that she definitely knew.

Being a doctor working clinical hours and a mother of two teenager boys, her schedule was very busy. On the exercise front, she was being consistent. She generally got up early to get in her workouts, which were mostly outdoor boot-camp style HIIT workouts and a lot of body weight and core work, with easy workouts on Friday and Sunday.

Nutritionally, she was doing okay, but fell into a common trap for busy women: backloading the day. Though she squeezed in a bite or two during the day, it wasn't enough, and come dinnertime she was super hungry. So while she was cooking she'd have a glass or two of wine and some carrots and hummus, trying to mitigate her hunger until the meal was ready. She also was low on protein and, in general, was in a state of low energy availability (LEA). Judy really needed to develop specific eating habits for before and after her training, using meal timing as training fuel (so she's not relying on coffee and protein shakes). Doing this would give her the energy she needed to perform and recover, and kick her out of this state of LEA (and the muscle loss, fat gain, and thyroid dysfunction and fatigue that follows), even if she doesn't fully fulfill her calorie needs for the rest of the day.

Having proper breakfasts and lunches would create more opportunities for her to get more diverse, whole foods into her diet and improve her gut microbiome, giving her healthy, even energy levels. Her new priority was getting 40 grams of protein at every meal.

I also wanted her to focus on true recovery and sleep. She woke up very early every day, even on Friday, her easy day. Saturday and Sunday she could sleep in a bit, but she often got up early anyway to try to get some work in before the day started. She wasn't not getting enough parasympathetic (rest and digest) activation to help her body reduce the cortisol load.

Finally, I suggested trying some adaptogens for four months to see how that might help mitigate some of her vasomotor symptoms (like the hot flashes), sleep disruption, and brain fog, before she committed to MHT.

HER NEW ROUTINE

Here's how her new schedule looks after our makeover:

MONDAY: Sleep in! She now starts off the week with a little sleep in the bank and has a bit of a recovery day. She has clinic from 8:30 a.m. to 3:30 p.m. If she feels like it, afterward she can go for a 25 to 30 minute run with some short 20-second intervals.

TUESDAY: Boot camp and grand rounds. She takes a breakfast smoothie so she can drink that on the way to grand rounds, for recovery and to keep her from getting hungry during the meeting. Then she has a small breakfast afterward. During the day she snacks on carrots and hummus here and there until lunch.

WEDNESDAY: 12-hour clinic day. We work in strategic snacking so she's not subsisting on coffee and protein shakes. She brings mini meals that include fruits and veggies and protein. That way she's building a healthy gut microbiome and keeps amino acids in her circulation to maintain her muscles. Then we add a 30 minute yoga session to the end of her day to activate her parasympathetic nervous system and put her in deep relaxation before bed.

THURSDAY: Same as Tuesday. Boot camp, smoothie, and a mini meal between patients. Then a 15 minute break midday for lunch. After work she can go for an easy chill run or a little hike just to blow off the stress of the day, keeping the rating of perceived exertion (RPE) at 6 or less.

FRIDAY: Swimming . . . a little later. She pushes the swim with her friend to 7 instead of 6 a.m. to allow more sleep. Coffee and breakfast afterward, then off to clinic. She has dinner at 7 p.m. and relaxes for the evening.

SATURDAY: CrossFit morning, but now she has a substantial breakfast at 7 a.m. when she gets up. Then she has two hard-boiled eggs and a handful of almonds on her way home to get some protein in circulation right away.

SUNDAY: She alternates between taking Sunday off and chilling with her family or all of them going on a short, easy run or some other low-intensity activity.

She started using ashwagandha and schisandra in the morning. She implemented good sleep hygiene habits, winding down before bed with some mindfulness and less screen time. She also started using a Whoop band to track her sleep and recovery so she could see the results of her changes.

THE RESULTS

After five months, she lost nearly 20 pounds and dropped her body fat by 5 to 6 percent. She was able to reduce her vasomotor symptoms to one hot flash every few days. She improved her sleep quality and deep wave sleep. She's feeling stronger and fitter and has more energy. She's very happy to have reached her goals without substantially changing her life or taking hormone therapy.

STOP THE LEAKS

Your gut is lined with a thin, protective mucosal barrier that works as a two-way gatekeeper: important nutrients are allowed out into circulation while nasty germs are locked in so they can't enter your bloodstream. Strenuous exercise, especially in hot conditions, can make the gut more permeable.

Anti-inflammatories such as NSAIDs (ibuprofen, acetaminophen, and naproxen sodium) and aspirin can make a leaky gut worse. These medications work by blocking the production of certain prostaglandins (hormone-like substances) that promote inflammation. There are also prostaglandins that protect the lining of the stomach and intestines, however, and NSAIDs decrease the production of them too. With fewer prostaglandins, the protective mucosa of the gut is eroded, and that leads in turn to a condition aptly called "leaky gut," which paves the way for harmful bacteria to get into circulation, interfere with healthy kidney function, and make it easier to get dehydrated. Leaky gut also can hinder recovery. Steer clear of those NSAIDs. Eat an anti-inflammatory diet and use naturally anti-inflammatory adaptogens instead.

For extra protection, you can buffer your gut before a hard exercise session with a calcium supplement. If you do not have issues with irritable bowel syndrome (IBS), using calcium carbonate can help maintain intestinal integrity and prevent muscle cramping. Take a peppermint Tums about 20 minutes before heading out the door. The calcium works with neuromuscular contractions and muscle metabolism, and the carbonate helps keep the junctions of the intestinal cells together, reducing endotoxin release and the ensuing symptoms.

If you do have chronic IBS issues, you will want to use chewable calcium citrate. The difference is that the citrate reduces the inflammation that invokes leaky gut, whereas the carbonate just helps keep the junctions intact. You can pop some additional Tums to help slow down GI distress during high-intensity sessions such as intervals or a race, and especially during ultra-style events. Selene used to struggle with nausea during her ultra-endurance events, which hurt her performance not only in the moment but also down the line, because it became a challenge to take in calories. Taking a Tums every couple of hours made her gut—and her race experience—much happier.

There are also a few products, such as Goodgut, that contain polyphenol-based prebiotics that can help maintain the lining of the gut. By reducing the erosion of the gut mucosa, you maintain the natural barrier for a longer period of time, since it can erode in as little as 30 minutes. These products work especially well when the gut is stressed from increased body heat, low oxygen, and low blood circulation during exercise. You can use this type of product each morning of a taper week to significantly improve your gut integrity going into a big event.

GUT BACTERIA EXERCISE BENEFITS AND RISKS

Moderate exercise is good for gut health. Key benefits include:

- Enriched gut microbiome diversity—the cornerstone of good gut health and well-being
- Better bacterial balance from improvements to the Bacteroidetes-to-Firmicutes ratio—the key to maintaining a healthy weight and reducing the risk of accumulating deep belly fat
- A stronger gut barrier to help prevent leaky gut
- Stimulation of bacteria activity that improves overall health, such as better brain health and lower risk of cancer

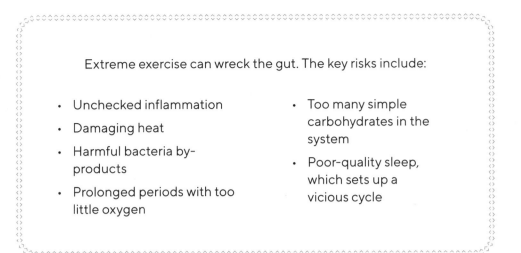

Extreme exercise can wreck the gut. The key risks include:

- Unchecked inflammation
- Damaging heat
- Harmful bacteria by-products
- Prolonged periods with too little oxygen
- Too many simple carbohydrates in the system
- Poor-quality sleep, which sets up a vicious cycle

HYDRATING FOR A HEALTHY MICROBIOME

How you hydrate during exercise also impacts the health of your gut. Fluids need a certain osmolality (concentration of salt and sugar) to be transported from the gut into your bloodstream. That's why plain water isn't great for quick hydration—it just sits there. For fast absorption, the fluid you drink needs to have an osmolality that is lower than your blood plasma (the watery part of your blood) so that your body can pull the fluid into circulation, where it can help keep you cool and hydrated.

I recommend using a sports drink that is relatively low in carbs, about 3 to 3.5 percent carbs (or 7 grams per 8 ounces). That is just enough sugar (ideally dextrose and sucrose) to activate all the gut transporters without overloading any of them, and enough sodium to facilitate optimum hydration but not so much that the fluid stalls out in the gut. These lower-carb drinks also help protect the gut microbiome from the harmful effects of too much sugar. This is particularly important when your gut is already compromised during exertion.

Also look for natural products without artificial flavors, colors, or hidden fillers that can cause microbe imbalances and aggravate the gut. The more you exercise, the more important this is. Even if you eat microbiome-friendly foods during daily life, you can undo that during intense exercise by drinking multiple bottles of fluids filled with lots of sugar and other ingredients that wreak havoc on a healthy gut microbiome . . . and that in turn is counterproductive to all your hard work.

GUT-WRECKING BOMBS

We can drink kombucha and fill our plates with polyphenol-rich foods, but we can't expect our happy and healthy microbiomes to withstand the assault that many of us launch on our gut each day. Here are some of the most common gut microbiome bombs that women take in on a regular basis and how to protect against them.

ANTIBIOTICS: The name says it all—*anti*-biotic. These drugs are without question an essential part of our modern medical arsenal and have improved and extended lives worldwide. They are also being horribly abused and overused. According to a Centers for Disease Control (CDC) estimate, about half of all antibiotics prescribed are unnecessary or prescribed inappropriately. If you have a cold, sore throat, or other upper respiratory infection, chicken soup (with plenty of garlic) and rest is the way to go. Spare your gut flora the decimation caused by antibiotics and only take them when absolutely, positively necessary.

ARTIFICIAL SWEETENERS: Research suggests that artificial sweeteners alter your gut bacteria in ways that produce glucose intolerance. This intolerance usually develops when your body can't cope with heavy sugar loads in your diet, setting the stage for obesity and metabolic diseases like diabetes. The development of glucose intolerance may be one reason why people who drink lots of diet soda are actually more likely to be overweight despite taking in less sugar and fewer calories.

PROCESSED FOODS: Refined, sugary foods cause an explosion of Firmicutes in the gut. When this type of bacteria takes over your gut, weight gain typically follows.

9

EAT ENOUGH!

Stop dieting for good . . . seriously.

When I wrote my first book, *ROAR*, I devoted a lot of space to maintaining a healthy body composition and optimum performance by emphasizing energy availability—eating enough to fuel your exercise. Many active women simply do not eat enough to support their training and recovery. Ultimately, both their performance and their health suffer the consequences.

This is an issue that women struggle with their entire lives, and one of the biggest problems I see among my active clientele, especially as they reach menopause and see their body composition changing. They come to me because their training isn't working like it used to and they're gaining weight. So they cut way back on their food intake and that makes matters worse. Now their body is in conservation and survival mode.

There's a name for this: low energy availability, or LEA. It happens when your energy expenditure routinely exceeds your energy intake, so your body does not have enough energy available to support all the physiological functions you need to maintain optimal health.

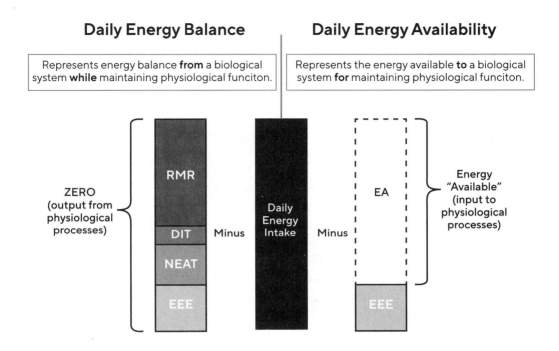

Daily Energy Balance

Represents energy balance **from** a biological system **while** maintaining physiological funciton.

Daily Energy Availability

Represents the energy available **to** a biological system **for** maintaining physiological funciton.

ZERO (output from physiological processes)

RMR

DIT

NEAT

EEE

Minus

Daily Energy Intake

Minus

EA

EEE

Energy "Available" (input to physiological processes)

In active women, LEA can result in a condition called relative energy deficiency in sport, or RED-S, which can lead to serious consequences like brittle bones and increased risk for heart disease. It's easy to identify when premenopausal women slip into this state: they stop having periods. You need enough energy to maintain healthy hormonal function, and when you have too little energy intake to meet your needs for too long, your hormones don't function properly and menstruation stops.

Identifying RED-S is harder in perimenopausal women, who may be having irregular periods, and in postmenopausal women, who obviously are no longer menstruating. We no longer have this big red (literally) flag warning us, "Whoa, you're not fueling properly." That's a problem, because RED-S can be extremely detrimental in menopausal women. Your thyroid function and bone formation start to be disrupted after just four days in low energy availability. Stay in that state too long and you can end up with extreme fatigue and thyroid dysfunction that is difficult to turn around.

Unless LEA/RED-S is identified and addressed, it also sets women up for a vicious, worsening cycle, because one of the first things that happens when the body isn't getting the energy it needs is that it starts increasing body fat. Without enough energy to perform basic functions (let alone your long runs or strength workouts), your endocrine system signals for your body to start breaking down muscle (which demands a lot of energy just to maintain itself) and to store more fat, so you have a reserve of energy. Our bodies are hardwired for survival. If you're not eating enough while you're working hard, your body assumes that you're in a situation where there's not enough food—so it stores all the energy it can to help you survive.

The next thing that happens is that your power declines. You've lost some muscle. You've stored some fat. And now your body is further conserving energy by lowering your metabolic output. Most women interpret this as a sign that they aren't training hard enough or that they're eating too much. So they try to train harder and eat less, making matters worse.

NAIL YOUR ENERGY AVAILABILITY

What should an active woman in her menopausal years be doing to maintain healthy energy availability? It starts with understanding metabolism, which has been shrouded in mystery to the point of being an ancient religion at this point.

Your "metabolism" is simply your daily energy expenditure. It is all the calories you burn in a day. Your metabolism is broken down into three parts:

BASAL METABOLIC RATE (BMR): Your BMR is the energy you burn just staying alive. Every cell of your body requires energy. You need energy to remodel bone, maintain muscle, and keep your brain function, immune system, hormone production, and other processes humming along. Your BMR accounts for about 60 to 80 percent of your metabolism.

THERMIC EFFECT OF FOOD (TEF): Digesting and processing food takes energy. About 10 percent of your daily energy expenditure is in the form of TEF.

ACTIVE METABOLISM: The rest of your daily energy expenditure is physical activity, whether that is puttering around the house or banging out a WOD at the CrossFit box. Obviously, the more energy you're using to exercise, the higher your energy demands.

When you have insufficient energy intake to meet your energy demand, you are left with too little energy reserve for all those important metabolic functions. As a result, your thyroid activity dims and your resting metabolic rate drops. Your cortisol becomes even more elevated, you develop resistance to growth hormone, and your hunger hormone (ghrelin) levels increase while your satiety hormone (leptin) levels decrease.

It can become very difficult to bring your metabolic rate back up when you hit this point. Despite what you may have read in mainstream magazines, you can't "boost" your metabolism with coffee and hot peppers. Those give it a little bump, but a temporary one. Coffee and peppers can't help you regain a healthy resting metabolic rate.

Notice that I've made no mention of calories. "Calories in, calories out" tells us nothing about how LEA and RED-S develop because, as we'll talk about in a bit, you can be eating all the calories you need but still are not getting the right amount of energy. Why? Because of *when* you eat your food. So many women "bookend" their calories during the day. They have a bit of food in the morning, do a training session, maybe have a recovery snack or meal, then go through the day without eating much until they get home. Then they have a big dinner and snack before bed, often with the idea of helping fuel the next morning's workout. This pattern keeps your body in a state of breakdown: you are not giving your body the fuel it needs *when it needs it*, which is in and around the times of training stress. Thus, your body is getting the same message ("I'm not getting enough fuel") regardless of whether you're eating enough in a 24-hour period to meet your calorie/macro needs. Likewise, women often eat too little—often *very* little—on recovery days, thinking, *Oh,*

I don't need food since I'm not exercising. But the body is trying to recover! It needs food.

Often women end up in LEA because they are deliberately restricting their food intake, but not always. Sometimes women inadvertently end up with LEA because they start performing more high-intensity exercise, but since they're working out for a relatively short amount of time, it doesn't register that they need to eat more to support that harder training. They may not feel as hungry right away because their appetite is blunted by the intense exercise. So they go about their day as usual and then end up in a hole.

You also need to layer in the effects of the menopause transition. Estrogen can lead to reduced food intake and meal size. That's because it modulates a gene known as KISS1, which is expressed to stimulate the kisspeptin neurons (more on those in a bit) in certain sections of the hypothalamus that mute appetite and reduce cravings for fat. Ghrelin, the appetite hormone that rises during starvation and falls after a meal (aka the "hunger hormone"), and estrogen have an interesting relationship; estrogen can downplay the brain's perception of hunger by reducing the sensitivity of ghrelin receptors. Now leptin, the other appetite hormone that decreases during energy restriction (aka the "satiety hormone") is stimulated by estrogen and insulin. That may cause perimenopausal women—depending on their estrogen status—to just not have the same appetite signals to eat or stop eating. Once estrogen is gone, postmenopausal women are not experiencing the same appetite suppression because now ghrelin is unopposed and leptin is bottoming out.

Research does show, however, that healthy, older, postmenopausal women, on average, often don't meet their energy needs, especially when it comes to protein. One study found that postmenopausal women, on average, take in protein at the rate of 1.1 grams per kilogram per day, which is *well* below the amount that active or athletic postmenopausal women need, and that about 25 percent consumed less than the minimum recommended daily allowance. (Notably, those in the low protein group also had higher body fat and fat-to-lean body mass ratio than those who consumed a higher protein diet.)

As you can see in the chart, you can get into a low energy state from either side—eating too little food or training too hard. Your goal is to have energy intake that meets your energy demands. It is in this space—and this is important—that you start losing weight if you have excess fat stores to lose. That sounds counterintuitive. Many athletes have it in their heads that eating less and training more equals weight loss. That's the message for the more sedentary general population; most people are not actually exercising much and are generally consuming too much energy. This is *not* the case for active people who are doing lots of exercise. For you, eating less and training more can lead to a low energy state.

How do you know if you are staying in that healthy energy availability state, or if you're drifting into the red on either side, when you no longer have a menstrual cycle to tell you, "Hey, wait a second, back off and fuel more effectively"? You have to be on the lookout for other signals that your energy availability is dwindling.

LEA IN PERI/MENOPAUSAL ATHLETES

Matching Energy Intake with Energy Demand

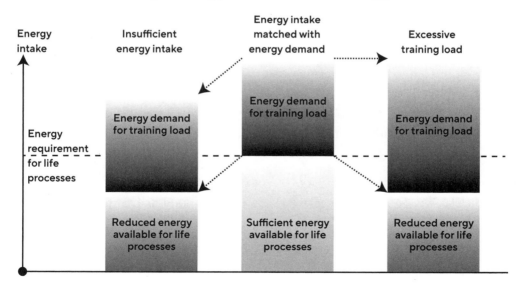

Here are some telltale signs to keep on your radar. Note that these are signs that trainers and coaches have traditionally chalked up to "overtraining." But very often they're actually a sign of underfueling and an indicator low energy availability.

DECREASED TRAINING RESPONSE: One of the first signs of lower energy availability is that your performance plateaus or decreases. You can't hit your wattage. You have less strength and power. Your heart rate is off. You're not recovering well.

DIMINISHING BONE HEALTH: Stress reactions and fractures are a major warning sign of low energy availability.

DECREASED IMMUNITY: You're more prone to infection. If you're starting to pick up every cold and every virus, your immune system is depressed.

INCREASE IN GUT DISTRESS: This one can be tricky for women because it can mimic other symptoms of the hormonal fluctuation that many women experience. But LEA also can cause IBS symptoms: bloating, gassiness, nausea, and generally not feeling well after eating. The problem is that your gut microbiome is off from the chronic inflammation that happens when your body is under stress from not having enough energy to perform all of its functions.

WORSENING COORDINATION: Without the energy you need, you are more fatigued, which impairs your cognition, reaction time, and coordination.

CHRONIC HANGRINESS: Low energy availability puts you in a state of perpetual "hangriness." You are going to be more irritable, anxious, and depressed. Your hunger cues may be gone at this point, so you don't even know that you're hangry. Or you may feel really hungry at odd times, like when you're out running errands or when it's time for bed. We also are finding out that women in LEA are often hypoglycemic through the night, which makes them wake up frequently, which of course, does not help anyone's mood!

When you start experiencing all these symptoms, you are at risk for developing full-on RED-S, a state where every system in your body is affected by low energy availability.

How do you fix LEA or get out of RED-S? By shrinking the gap between what your body requires and what you're putting in. Ideally, I'd recommend that you stop all formal training for three to four weeks while your body recovers. But I am a realist and realize that women have many different reasons to train beyond preparing for an event. (For most of us, in fact, that is at the bottom of the list!) Women train for stress relief, as a social outlet, and for their mental well-being. So it's fine to maintain a bit of training, but you want to bring down the total volume of exercise while maintaining a few short, high-intensity sessions and increasing your fueling during and around your workouts (when your body needs the energy most).

Remember, it is not about the total number of calories you eat in a day, but *when* you eat them that matters the most here. Eating at the right times will help you reestablish the connection between energy in and energy out that gets you into the happy space where your mood, recovery, and performance are improving and you have good energy availability for your daily life as well as your workouts.

Remember, too, that your gut microbiome takes a beating when you slip into energy deficiency for too long. Some of the anxiety and depression that you can experience from low energy availability is driven by the bacteria in your gut being in a state of hunger and waiting. They're like, "Hey, we need food too!" and are signaling to your brain that things are not okay, which in turn makes you feel not okay. Be sure to fuel yourself with microbiome-building foods, like a wide assortment of fruits and vegetables, while you are increasing your energy intake.

NEXT LEVEL MENOPAUSE MAKEOVER:
A RUNNER GETS HER GROOVE BACK

JANE,* 48, came to me after losing her joy of running to sudden weight gain, soreness, and general menopausal malaise. All she really wanted was to get her running groove back.

GENERAL ASSESSMENT

Jane loves to run. She's never been interested in racing. She likes to mix it up with swimming and rock climbing and other fun activities. But her transition into menopause, which started with hot flashes when she was 46, was stealing her joy. By the time she came to see me two years later, she had gained 20 pounds despite not doing anything differently in her training or nutrition.

At that point she was 132 pounds (she's 5'4") and 28 percent body fat, which is certainly in the healthy range, but was a bit outside of the athletic fitness range she had previously been in, and a little more weight than she typically carried on her small frame. When she started gaining weight, she did what millions of women do—and what she'd read about in running magazines—trained more and ate less, thinking the problem was with her "calories in versus calories out." Despite restricting calories, she continued to lose muscle and gain fat. She was also getting stress reactions, which are not full-on stress fractures, but painful bone bruises, especially in her feet and lower legs. She started feeling drained on most days. Though she could push through some workouts, she was sometimes skipping the last part of workouts and lagging behind in her running group, which she used to be leading. On her longer days, she started having a lot of GI issues. It was all really demotivating.

Unfortunately, her mindset of "calories in versus calories out" was really just promoting fatigue because she was slogging through workouts under fueled. This put her in a catabolic state—where she's eating into her muscles—as she's cutting calories and exercising fasted. That increases her cortisol and doesn't give her the fuel she needs to perform, and makes it harder to recover.

I want her to start fueling her workouts appropriately and eat real food. When she has a morning session, I want her to have a piece of toast with some almond butter beforehand. Afterward, I want her to have a bowl of yogurt with some fruit and nuts when she gets home. Splitting breakfast fuels both ends of her training without loading her up on ultra-processed sport foods that perturb the microbiome, which can increase fat storage. Because she's been relying on processed foods for so long, we also add some spirulina for iron, hemp and chia and flax seeds for plant-based proteins and fats and more fiber, all with the goal of building that gut microbiome diversity, which helps with estrogen metabolism and fatigue, as well as mitigating those GI issues.

We want to make her more injury- and stress-resilient to prevent the stress reactions she's been having, so we add a lifting program to build lean muscle and bone mass. We also include stretching and mobility work and adjust her schedule to make sure she's getting the sleep she needs.

HER NEW ROUTINE

Here's how her new schedule looks after our makeover:

MONDAY: Hard training day. Instead of training early, she sleeps in and does a heavy lifting session at lunch. She does 3 to 4 sets of 5 reps of heavy squats and deadlifts along with some core work. Then she does a 20 minute treadmill session with increasing gradients, which is like her hill training, but very specific, improving her running mechanics. She's in and out of the gym in an hour.

TUESDAY: Super easy day. She does a walk/jog workout, keeping her RPE at 4 or 5 on a 1 to 10 scale.

WEDNESDAY: Morning track session. She fuels like she did on Monday with almond butter toast and a latte. She has some hydration drink and raisins on the side of the track to keep her energy up during the second half of the session. Then she eats overnight oats in the car as she is driving to work.

THURSDAY: Gym day, moderately hard. Her legs are a bit tired from Wednesday's track workout. She goes to the gym and does a few heavy lifts with a very short plyometric session (such as 10 to 12 box jumps and plyometric push-ups) to finish. It's short and sharp and the whole session is 40 minutes.

FRIDAY: Garage training day. She can do an easy run and then do a circuit of kettlebell swings, lunges, and box jumps. This is all just to keep her mobility and functional strength and fitness to support her running.

SATURDAY: Super easy run. Just a pleasure cruise to keep her aerobic capacity.

SUNDAY: Easy play day. Go hiking, rock climbing, or skip exercise-related activity all together and take a cooking class. If she feels tight or like she wants to move, she can do her yoga.

She followed the schedule for a few months and we adjusted it along the way, because she really got into the lifting and wanted to focus more on that, with less on the cardiovascular training.

As she pivoted her training routine toward more resistance training and lifting, the volume of her training went down as the intensity went up. The stress reactions went away (as she gained bone density) and she became stronger, better fueled, and more resilient. She was also sleeping better, which helps with recovery.

On the diet front, we made sure she ate real foods and carbohydrates around her training early in the day and then tapered them down over the course of the afternoon, because she didn't need them.

THE RESULTS

After six months, she lost 10 to 12 pounds and brought her body fat into the athletic range. She didn't lose the 20 pounds she wanted, but as I explained to her, when you're increasing your lean mass with heavy lifting, the scale isn't telling the whole story. I also think this is a healthier weight for her overall—in the years before her menopause-induced weight gain she had been forcing herself into an artificially underweight state because she thought that's what she should be doing to be a runner.

It took some work to shift her from that "lighter is better" mindset many runners have, but in the end, she admitted that it was impossible to deny that she was feeling and performing better without counting calories and denying herself the fuel she needed.

TRAINING GAINS ARE MADE IN THE KITCHEN

There's a saying that abs are made in the kitchen. It's a nod to the fact that all the training in the world won't yield the results you're looking for without the proper nutrition to support it. This was most definitely the case with a triathlete I worked with who was in chronic LEA. She would eat a small bit before some of her training sessions and a protein drink after, but her overall calorie intake was around 1,800 to 2,000 a day when she was regularly expending 2,500 to 2,800 a day.

I finally convinced her to start gradually increasing her food intake (mostly carbohydrates) over the course of four weeks. At the end of the fourth week, her functional threshold power (the maximum amount of power you can maintain for about an hour) had gone up, as if she had just done a heavy block of FTP (functional threshold power) intensive training, yet she was only following the low total volume recovery mode that I recommend for LEA athletes.

THE PERIL OF POPULAR DIET TRAPS

One very common way that women slip into a state of LEA and RED-S is by following trendy diets like intermittent fasting and ketosis. It can be incredibly difficult to maintain healthy energy availability if you're following a rigid, super-restrictive diet plan. But, again, when women start to gain weight, this is often the first thing they try.

It's completely understandable. All the magazines, including ones dedicated to sport, write glowingly about various diet fads. They're everywhere on the internet. Social media influencers or Fitspo folks (who, by the way, generally use filters and take dozens of shots to get that perfectly "effortless" look) push them on their channels. Don't feel bad if you've been swept up in one (or more!) of these fads in the past. But now I'm going to give you some ammunition for resisting the most popular diet trends often marketed to peri- and postmenopausal women.

INTERMITTENT FASTING IS NOT YOUR FRIEND

Intermittent fasting is the practice of restricting your calorie intake to a shortened window. There are many variations on the practice. Some people restrict calories to a super-short four-hour window, basically eating one meal a day. Others extend it to an eight-hour window or, at the outer limit, twelve hours.

Fasting has a long history of being practiced for religious reasons, and I won't dispute it as a spiritual practice. But fasting for health purposes, especially fasting among active *women* for health purposes? That I will dispute . . . and discourage.

The basic health premise behind intermittent fasting is that if you deprive your body of food for long periods, it will lower your insulin levels and burn your stored fat for fuel. Proponents believe that by putting the body under this stress, it is forced to adapt in healthy ways, much as it does under exercise stress.

Much of the original fasting and health research came out in the mid-1930s, a time characterized by war and widespread economic hardship. Scientists wanted to see what would happen to people's health if they restricted their food intake for economic reasons. As was standard practice, they only included men in their human studies. They found that restricting calories by about 20 percent was beneficial for health. Follow-up research (again on men) confirmed that calorie restriction leads to increases in telomere length. (Telomeres are a region of DNA that shortens over time and acts as a biological marker for aging.) Calorie restriction also appeared to increase autophagy—the body's way of cleaning out damaged cells in order to regenerate newer, healthier cells.

More recently, medical scientists have been investigating intermittent fasting as a way to help people with obesity. These studies have been done on people who are reflective of the general population: they are overweight or obese and have unhealthy blood lipids and blood glucose levels.

Generally speaking, the men in these studies did really well with calorie restriction. Regardless of age, they had improved insulin sensitivity, so they were at lower risk for diabetes; they had lower LDL and triglyceride levels so their cardiovascular health improved; they had better autophagy, increasing their body's ability to clean up cellular debris; and they had lower levels of oxidative stress, so their cells were protected from free radical damage. They scored better on memory tests, showing that even their brains worked better. It's easy to look at that research and think, *Wow, that's fantastic!*

Now let's look at data from the women in the research. When you look at sedentary women, there was no benefit for insulin sensitivity from calorie restriction. In fact, women who had high blood sugar and were on the cusp of becoming diabetic actually saw a worsening in their insulin sensitivity and blood sugar. On the plus side, women saw an increase in their good HDL levels, but there was no shift in their LDL or triglyceride levels. Unlike men, women had minimal, if any, improvement in autophagy. And they actually had increased oxidative stress. Worse, fasting had adverse affects on their endocrine system. So their thyroid function slowed down and took their metabolism with it. As a woman, your body will fight to preserve energy when you start fasting.

This picture gets worse for women who exercise. If you exercise on top of fasting—which is what many women try to do to lose weight—all of these negative effects become amplified. That's pretty much the opposite of what you're looking for as a menopausal woman struggling to maintain a healthy metabolism and good metabolic and cardiovascular health.

Now, if you take out the fasting and just add the exercise? Everything improves. You reduce cardiovascular risk factors. You increase autophagy. You lower your inflammation and oxidative stress. Your endocrine system functions better. So all in all, fasting is not good for women, especially exercising women.

JUST SAY NO TO KETO

The other diet trend that many menopausal women are tempted by is the ketogenic diet. The "keto" diet is extremely low-carb, limiting intake to fewer than 50 grams of carbs a day, or the amount in one small apple and a cup of oatmeal. Instead, you get the bulk of your calories from a lot of fat (more than 60 percent of your intake) and moderate amounts of protein.

Without carbohydrates supplying blood glucose, the keto diet forces your body to produce energy by breaking down stored fat molecules called ketones in the liver; this process is called ketogenesis, which is where the name comes from.

The premise is that since menopausal women have higher amounts of visceral fat and insulin resistance, ketogenesis will help burn more fat and turn that around. On paper it sounds good.

As is so often the case, the original research on the ketogenic diet was done on men, specifically, metabolically unhealthy men who had obesity and/or had diabetes. The research was designed to see if they could get their blood sugar under control and lose weight quickly on a ketogenic diet. It worked in that population.

It also works okay in sedentary women. In the small amount of research that's been done on postmenopausal women, the keto diet does reduce weight gain, improve insulin sensitivity, and reduce cravings and food moods (hangriness).

The problem comes when people take research findings from sedentary, largely unhealthy people and apply them to an active, exercising population, especially women. Active women are told, "Hey, if you do this diet and increase your fat burning, you don't have to use as much carbohydrate. That means you can go longer, farther, and burn more body fat while you exercise." That does sound great.

But what this research doesn't show is how ketogenesis affects women who are training and exercising. It doesn't work the same way for women as it does for men. Your body uses carbohydrates to kick-start fat burning. So even if you're primed to use fat for fuel—and women, more so than men, already are primed to use more fat as fuel—you still need carbohydrates to access your fat-burning metabolism. Denying your body carbohydrates during exercise is a huge stress. Research shows the keto diet has an unfavorable effect on muscle fatigue on women. Research shows markers of bone remodeling are impaired after a short-term low-carb, high-fat diet. Neither is good for menopausal women!

And let's not forget kisspeptin, mentioned earlier. Kisspeptin is a small protein produced by your neurons that helps regulate reproductive function and plays a significant role in maintaining healthy blood sugar, appetite, and body composition. Women are more sensitive to changes in kisspeptin than men, which makes sense when you consider its role in reproductive function. When your brain perceives nutrient deficiency, especially a deficiency of carbohydrates, there is a marked reduction in kisspeptin stimulation, which not only increases your appetite but also reduces your sensitivity to insulin (and we already know this is an associated side effect of perimenopause). As a result, you feel hungrier, don't get a strong signal that you're full, and store more fat.

What happens when you layer exercise stress on top of the stress of denying your body an important fuel source? Stress hormones like cortisol rise even higher, which is bad for menopausal women, who, as we know, already have increased cortisol levels. As you keep increasing that stress, it keeps your sympathetic drive high and reduces your ability to relax. Your thyroid activity is depressed. Your body starts storing more belly fat. And worse, your risk for fatty liver disease increases.

The bottom line here is that anything that drives your cortisol up is a big warning flag telling you to step back, stay away, and say, "Not for me."

THE POSITIVE BENEFITS OF PLANT-BASED EATING

Let's end on a diet trend that *is* beneficial for menopausal women: plant-based eating, which is usually thought of as a vegetarian or vegan diet. But in our context, "plant-based" refers to eating mostly food from plant sources, with small amounts of high-quality animal products.

Generally speaking, the research on plant-based eating in both sedentary and active women (and men) is very positive. People who follow a plant-based diet generally have lower BMI, lower body fat, improved blood lipid levels, and better blood sugar control. People who eat a wide variety of fruits and vegetables also have lower levels of inflammation, higher levels of antioxidants, and lower risks of cancer, diabetes, and heart disease. They also have better gut health, because plant foods enhance the diversity of the bacteria in the microbiome.

The gut health benefits are particularly pertinent for menopausal women, because, as the last chapter illustrated, the gut microbiome affects everything, including body composition, mood, and immunity. A healthy gut also may help relieve menopausal symptoms. A 2018 study published in *Maturitas* found that, among perimenopausal women, vegans reported fewer bothersome vasomotor symptoms like hot flashes and fewer physical symptoms as measured by the menopause-specific quality of life questionnaire than omnivores. Eating more vegetables and fewer animal foods was associated with a decrease in both types of symptoms.

The good news is that you don't have to be a strict, 100 percent vegan to reap benefits. If you eat some animal products but make fruit, vegetables, and other plant foods the center of your meals, you can still get the benefits of a plant-based diet.

10

FUELING FOR
THE MENOPAUSE TRANSITION

*These smart food choices can ease symptoms
and improve health and performance.*

J ust tell me what to eat!"
I cannot tell you how many times I've heard those words. We're so bombarded with confusing, conflicting messages (whether or not we're looking for them) on what we should and should not be eating that it's not surprising how overwhelming nutrition is for most people.

It gets worse once we reach our menopausal years. For some of us, this may be the first time we have felt at a loss as to what we should or shouldn't be eating because our bodies are changing seemingly overnight and what has worked for us up to this point appears to no longer be doing the job.

Adapting your diet to work with your changing physiology during this time is important not only for performance but also for your general health. Research shows that the average woman's deep belly fat (the inflammatory, health-wrecking kind) increases 44 percent during menopause. This is why you're three times more likely to develop metabolic syndrome—increased blood pressure, high blood sugar, excess belly fat, and unhealthy lipid and triglyceride levels—after menopause than before.

As your sex hormones fluctuate, decline, and eventually flatline, your metabolism changes dramatically. You are more likely to become insulin-resistant and to have elevated blood sugar, so your relationship with carbohydrates has to change. You lose the sex hormones that drive muscle development, so you need to ramp up your protein and eat it at the right times to maintain your lean mass. The form of estrogen that dominates your circulation right now, estrone (E1), is one and a half to five times less potent than estradiol (E2), the "typical" estrogen we talk about. Your testosterone is also dropping. Exercise helps, of course. But it's not enough.

Obviously, working one-on-one with a dietitian is the only way to get fully personalized advice to meet your specific needs. I can't tell whether you have, for example, a history of iron deficiency, or nut allergies, or hereditary issues with cholesterol. What I can—and will—do here, however, is tell you in broad brush strokes how much energy you need, what your macronutrient intake should look like, and how to proportion your plate for your best health and performance during menopause and beyond.

FIRST: EAT ENOUGH!

I'm going to keep drilling that one in, because, for so many women, the number-one mistake they make is not eating enough. They've read in some women's magazine that they should be eating 1,200 to 1,500 calories a day—which can easily be 1,000 calories less than they need—and that number has stuck in their minds.

Here are the facts: 1,500 calories is the *bare* minimum of what you need to be eating if you're simply sitting on the couch and existing. Here is a chart based on a woman who weighs 130 pounds (59 kilograms) and has a body composition of 21 percent fat. (Your healthy body fat range depends on your age, but broadly speaking, it is 19 to 32 percent for active adult women.)

GUIDELINES FOR DAILY INTAKE

Macros (does NOT include training food)	Active recovery (light activity days, rest day)	Moderate Training (HIIT, 60 to 120min moderate intensity)	Heavy Training (sessions/day, >2.5 hours hard aerobic, >4h moderate aerobic)
Menopausal Female			
CHO (2 to 3.5g/kg)	148	177	207
PRO (1.8 to 2.4g/kg)	130	136	142
FAT (1 to 1.3g/kg)	59	71	71
	Example Female		
Body Weight (in kg)	59.00		
% body fat (in decimal form: e.g. 35% is 0.35)	0.21		
Fat Mass	12.39		
Lean Mass	46.61		

These are baseline macronutrient guidelines to keep your body out of low energy availability (LEA) and to keep adapting to exercise stress. They do not include fueling in and around exercise. That's extra and essential. Use this as a reference point to get a general idea of your ideal energy intake. But don't get fixated on calories. I prefer that women pay more attention to their macronutrients and allow the appropriate calories to come naturally. Because what is most important about the food that you're fueling yourself with is its composition—whether it has the right balance of carbohydrate, protein, and fat.

YOUR MENOPAUSE MACROS

I want to put in a word about macros and weight loss. I am not a huge fan of tracking macros and calories, as this can lead down the path to a disconnect between what it means to nourish and fuel your body vs focus on the numbers to change body composition/lose weight. We know that with age, our needs change, but if we focus on real, whole foods, eating a wide variety of fresh produce, lean protein, and having a fun factor built in for wine, chocolate and so on, it balances out. Actually it becomes more important when you eat (see the next chapter on nutrient timing) at this time. But, I get it. There are those who want to track and want to know how much of what to eat; so here we go. Your optimum macronutrient mix changes once you hit menopause because, again, without your sex hormones, you become more carbohydrate-sensitive and have a harder time building and holding on to muscle. In general, you'll be eating a little less carbohydrate and a little more protein and fat than you might have in your younger years. As the chart shows, your needs change with activity. But at the very minimum, on a totally sedentary day, your macronutrients should look like this:

Carbohydrates: 2 grams per kilogram of body weight

Protein: 1.8 to 2 grams per kilogram of body weight, distributed evenly throughout meals

Fat: 1+ grams per kilogram of body weight

As you increase your activity from a light day with easy exercise (walking, yoga, or mobility work) to a day with a moderate level of activity (a HIIT session or one to two hours of cardio) to a heavy day (two-a-day sessions, more than two and a half hours of hard cardio, or more than four hours of any cardio), your energy needs go up in tandem with your activity level. Most of the time, women fall into that moderate activity category, for which they need each day, on average, 3 grams of carbohydrates per kilogram of body weight; 2 to 2.2 grams of protein per kilogram of body weight; and 1.2 grams of fat per kilogram of body weight.

So on that moderate training day, our 130-pound woman would be eating about 1,900 calories plus a snack during training, which takes her to about 2,000 calories. That's a far cry from what a lot of women eat. Note: If you are trying to lose weight, you can figure your macros toward your goal weight—but within reason! You want to make small adjustments, so you don't lose muscle and bone.

It's important to balance your macronutrients throughout the day, especially protein. Since your body responds best to a more even protein distribution throughout the day, try to get 30 grams of protein at each meal and 15 to 20 grams with your snacks. Aim for your biggest protein hit—about 30 to 40 grams—for right after you train.

SMART SWEETENERS

Many women are smartly trying to limit their intake of added sugars. Unfortunately, unscrupulous marketers take advantage of that effort and advertise their sweeteners as "healthy" because they're "natural." A perfect example of that is agave syrup. Agave syrup is highly processed and much higher in fructose than plain sugar. In fact, it's just the same as high-fructose corn syrup, so it's more likely to cause adverse health effects like belly fat.

Honey is a better option, because it contains polyphenols, which are antioxidants. Maple syrup is another good option. In fact, I often rate maple syrup as one of the best sweeteners because it is the least processed. It's just glucose and sucrose. If you're looking for one be-all-end-all sweetener, maple syrup is the way to go.

The quality of your carbohydrates is essential now. Meeting your carb needs with bagels and brownies is not going to cut it because your body needs fiber and nutrient-dense food to maintain your gut microbiome, manage your blood sugar, support your hormones, and supply even amounts of energy as your sex hormones slide. Some starchy carbs and whole grains are good when you need a dense source of carbs to fuel activity, but the bulk of your carbohydrates at this point should be coming from fruits and vegetables to help maintain healthy insulin levels, blood sugar, and overall health (more on that later). Winter squash and root vegetables like sweet potatoes, parsnips, and beets are excellent substitutions for breads and pastas because they're rich in fiber that builds up the gut microbiome and phytonutrients that fight disease.

Do not fall into the trap of worrying about the sugar in fruits and vegetables. Yes, they contain natural sugars like fructose, but those sugars are wrapped in fiber, which your gut microbiome needs. If you're worried about fluctuations in your blood sugar levels, you can pair your higher-glycemic-index fruits and veggies with nuts, cottage cheese, and other protein-rich foods that counteract some of the

WHAT TO EAT?

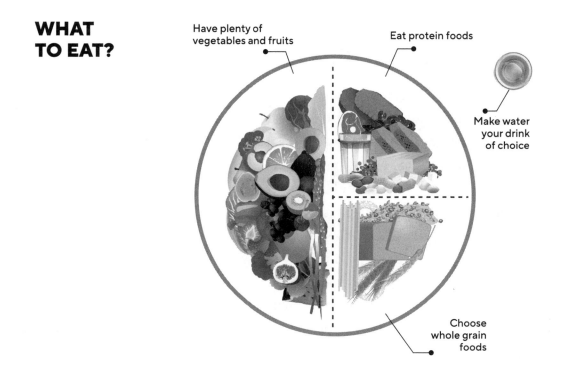

Have plenty of vegetables and fruits

Eat protein foods

Make water your drink of choice

Choose whole grain foods

blood glucose response. You also can save your starchy veggies for right after training, when your body is most responsive to restocking your glycogen stores.

The Active Menopause Plate shown before gives you an idea of the ideal proportions of the macronutrients you should be consuming. I realize, of course, that your meals will not always be neatly laid out on a plate, as they are here. Sometimes you have soup, stir-fries, wraps, or what have you. But this is a good visualization of the proportions of each macronutrient that should be present.

Half of every meal should be a variety of colorful fruits and vegetables. Think of these as the base of your meals. A quarter of your meal should come from protein foods, so any kind of lean meat like bison or organic beef, chicken, and fish; a mix of beans; tofu or tempeh; and/or eggs. The final quarter should be your whole grains and starches. Again, look to make these as fiber- and nutrient-dense as possible, so emphasize sprouted brown rice, black rice, quinoa, sprouted grain bread, and bean- or pulse-based pasta.

BROCCOLI AND BRUSSELS SPROUTS

You already know the usual reasons that cruciferous vegetables are good for you. They're rich in antioxidants, vitamins and minerals, and fiber. But for menopausal women they are especially important because they help manage your hormones.

Cruciferous vegetables like broccoli, cauliflower, kale, Brussels sprouts, and cabbage are particularly good for hormone management. When you eat cruciferous vegetables, your stomach acid breaks down one of their compounds called indole-3-carbinol to produce diindolylmethane (DIM). DIM affects your estrogen levels, specifically stimulating the production of a less potent, more beneficial form of estrogen known as 2-hydroxyestrone. DIM also blunts the effects of another, more potent form of estrogen called 16alpha-hydroxyestrone, which has been linked to an increased risk for breast and uterine cancer as well as fat gain. In addition, DIM helps block an enzyme known as aromatase from converting testosterone to estrogen, which is a good thing for your muscle maintenance needs.

DIM is such a beneficial compound for women that you can buy it in pill form as an over-the-counter supplement that purportedly supports estrogen metabolism, fights hot flashes, and helps with PMS symptoms. It's really just concentrated broccoli.

The more cruciferous vegetables you eat, the better your hormonal health and the lower your risk for increased abdominal fat accumulation. These vegetables are also very good for your gut microbiome because they provide a lot of prebiotic fiber.

As is typically the case with nutrients, getting them from food is better than getting them through a pill. We'll discuss DIM supplements in chapter 18. You may or may not decide to go that route, but you should most definitely make colorful produce, especially cruciferous vegetables, part of your daily diet. Pro tip: I realize that some women really dislike the bitterness of cruciferous vegetables. (A gene that makes some women "supertasters" increases bitterness perception.) If that's you, roasting your cruciferous veggies is the way to go. It brings out the natural sweetness and cuts the bitterness that often shines through in other cooking methods like steaming or even sautéing.

SKIP THE MULTIS

It's tempting to pop a multivitamin supplement to "cover your bases." But these pills have been broadly oversold and are generally not worth the money. What most people don't consider is that there are so many different vitamins and minerals in a multivitamin supplement that they can cancel each other out. For instance, a typical multivitamin has calcium and iron, which bind to each other, so both become inactive. Chances are good that your body also doesn't need most of the micronutrients in a multivitamin, so you end up with expensive urine as the excess is excreted. Moreover, research has failed to find any benefit behind multivitamin supplementation.

They don't improve your health. In fact, some research on older women has found an association between vitamin and mineral supplement use and *increased* mortality risk. Better to get your vitamins and minerals from real food, where they naturally exist alongside complementary nutrients that enhance their absorption.

PLANT-BASED PROTEIN SOURCES

Combining your heavy strength training with a big hit of protein is the best way to stimulate muscle protein synthesis and make the muscle you need. Getting a big dose of protein after you lift heavy sh*t also extends what is known as the anabolic window—the period of time when your body is most responsive to making muscle is up to four hours after a workout. If you do a hard, high-intensity workout, adequately dosing with protein afterward will drop the levels of your stress hormone cortisol, bring your body out of that muscle-eating catabolic state, and lengthen the window of time for developing lean mass.

For recovery purposes, you want to be sure you get that 30 to 40 grams within 30 minutes following a HIIT or strength training session. The same goes for any workout that lasts longer than an hour to 90 minutes, like a long ride or run. If you've just done a yoga class or some easy exercise that doesn't get your heart rate up high or break down muscle tissue, you can get the protein you need at your next meal. You don't have to worry about hitting that recovery window of 30 minutes.

Consuming enough protein will also help you maintain healthy blood pressure and can reduce menopause symptoms like hot flashes, fatigue, mood swings, and brain fog, because the various amino acids found in protein-rich foods are vital for the production of hormones and neurotransmitters and other building blocks for good menopausal health.

For example, the amino acid arginine helps with endothelial function (how well your blood vessels dilate and contract). Lysine prevents arginine from being absorbed, so you have more of it hanging around to help keep those blood vessels working their best. Leucine enhances muscle protein synthesis, so your workouts yield better results. It also blocks tryptophan in the brain, which reduces serotonin to healthy levels and helps prevent brain fog and central nervous system fatigue. When you ramp up your protein intake during your menopausal years, you have a bigger amino acid pool circulating in your system and have the ability to draw on the ones you need to keep all your systems functioning at a higher level.

Often when women hear how much protein they need now, their eyes kind of pop out of their head and I can almost hear them thinking, *How am I going to get that much protein?* Many of these women equate protein with meat, so naturally it might feel off-putting to contemplate putting that much more meat on their plate, even if they typically eat animal foods. Those who don't eat meat may wonder if they're going to have to switch to a carnivore diet. As a longtime plant-based athlete myself, that's the *last* thing I'd tell you to do! You can get plenty of protein from plant sources and just a small to moderate amount of animal food or meat in your diet. As you can see in the next chart, protein is found throughout the plant world in nuts and nut butters, oatmeal, seeds, spinach, and beans of all kinds. If you eat dairy, it's *very* easy to get ample protein with Greek yogurt, cottage cheese, eggs, and other cheeses.

Here are some great food choices for getting protein without meat or nuts.

WHAT ABOUT PROTEIN?

Aim for 1.8 to 2.4g of protein per kg of bodyweight per day spread throughout the day

Top Meatless Protein Sources:	Top Meatless (and Nut-Free) Protein Sources:
• Cauliflower (5g/per serving (180g)) • Broccoli (5g/per serving (180g)) • Seeds (6g per handful) • Spinach (5g per serving (180g)) • Nut butters (8g per 2 tbsp) • Beans (15g per serving (180g)) • Oatmeal (8g per cup) • Eggs (8g per egg) • Greek Yogurt (10g per 100g) • Nuts (8g per handful)	• California Roll (6g per 5 piece serving) • Sunflower Seed Butter (7g per 2 tbsp serving) • Milk, dairy or soy (8g per 1 cup) • Edamame, in pods (9g per 1 cup) • Whole grain crackers (3g per 15 cracker serving) • Vegetarian burger or "chicken" patty (9g) • Tofu (9g per 3 cup serving) • Cheese Tortellini (10g per ¾ cup serving) • Slice of cheese pizza (12g per slice from 14" pizza) • String Cheese (6g per stick) • Hummus (2g per 2 tbsp serving) • Broccoli (2g per ¾ cup serving) • Popcorn (2g per 2 cup serving) • Avocado (2g per half-avocado) • Roasted Chickpeas (5g per ¼ cup serving)

A SUPER-SMOOTHIE

Getting your daily dose of protein is super-easy if you have a blender. You can blend frozen cauliflower, fresh spinach and kale, Greek yogurt, and mixed seeds like hemp and chia for a protein-packed super-smoothie. And the cruciferous veggies give you a double menopause win.

KEEP PROTEIN POWDERS IN THEIR PLACE

Protein powders are convenient and can be great for quick recovery after a race or when it's tough to find real food. But I encourage you to save them for those circumstances and not make protein shakes your first stop for meeting your protein needs. Not only are they expensive, but they can be high in sugar and some contain fillers and other ingredients you don't need. (Some women also find that protein powders make them gassy.) Real food always comes in the right package with the right ingredients you need without the additives you don't.

When you do reach for protein powder, whey isolate powders are the best for bioavailability. The best vegan alternative is pea-protein isolate, as it is just on the cusp of the leucine amount needed. Mix in hemp or brown rice, and you've got a perfect alternative to whey isolate.

WINNING CARBOHYDRATE-PROTEIN COMBINATIONS

One way to get more protein while lowering your carbohydrates is to put more emphasis on foods that contain both, but in the ratios you're looking for. That's one of the benefits of legumes like beans, lentils, chickpeas, and peanuts, as well as seeds. You can get fiber and carbs along with a healthy hit of protein.

This chart shows other winning carbohydrate-protein combinations like nuts, yogurt, cottage cheese, and even some animal foods like eggs and certain shellfish.

HIGH-PROTEIN LOW-CARBOHYDRATE FOODS

Aim for 1.8 to 2.4g per kg of bodyweight per day spread throughout the day

Salmon 25.2g protein 0 carb/4 oz	Peanut butter 7g protein 6 carbs/2 Tbsp	Greek yogurt 12g protein 19 carbs/1 cup
Chicken 24.2g protein 0 carb/4 oz	Sliced cheese 6.8g protein .6 carbs/1 oz	Almonds 6g protein 6.1 carbs/1 oz
Shrimp 22.8g protein 0 carb/4 oz	Eggs 6.3g protein 4 carbs/1 large	Sunflower seeds 5.4g protein 6.8 carbs/1 oz
Turkey 22.2g protein 0 carb/4 oz	Cottage cheese 14.9g protein 9.6 carbs/1 cup	Walnuts 4.3g protein 3.9 carbs/1 oz
Peanuts 7.3g protein 4.5 carbs/1 oz	Scallops 13.7g protein 3.6 carbs/4 oz	Cream cheese .9g protein 8 carbs/1 Tbsp

One question that comes up among the menopausal women I work with is whether eating a diet that is higher in protein will increase their cancer risk. We know that as our sex hormones flatline, levels of insulin growth factor (IGF-1), which is responsible for cell growth and important for bone and muscle development, also decrease. There's evidence that eating a high-protein diet increases IGF-1, which sounds like a positive. But research also has linked higher levels of IGF-1 with tumor development, particularly breast, colorectal, and prostate cancer. Hence the concern.

Here again, though, we see the benefit of combining healthy exercise habits with good nutrition. Adding exercise to the mix modulates IGF-1 expression and minimizes the risk. Statistically speaking, eating a high-protein diet in combination with a regular exercise routine has been shown to carry a very, very low risk for developing any kind of cancer. Plus, you're not eating a protein-dominant diet here, but one that better balances carbohydrates and proteins to optimize your changing physiology.

FOCUS ON LEUCINE

The amino acid leucine is known as the "trigger" for muscle growth. In fact, leucine, isoleucine, and valine make up about one-third of your muscle tissue. High-intensity exercise, menopausal changes, and post-exercise recovery increase the metabolism of leucine and can make you catabolic (meaning you're breaking down muscle tissue). Taking leucine shuts down that catabolic process. The more leucine you get into your system, the faster your muscles are saturated with it, and the more quickly they get the signal to repair and grow.

Generally speaking, if you consume 35 to 40 grams of whole protein, the leucine content will be 3 to 4 grams. Good protein sources of leucine include chicken, legumes, beans, salmon, brown rice, beef, tuna, firm tofu, milk, ricotta cheese, chia and flax seeds, and eggs. As with protein in general, I do not recommend adding leucine powder to a smoothie or post-workout recovery drink. Your essential amino acids work together, so taking one in isolation is not effective. It also tastes pretty bad, so chances are you won't finish what you started once you mix leucine powder in there.

If you feel like you're lacking in amino acids, you can add fermented BCAA (branched-chain amino acids) supplements to your diet ("fermented" means they come from only plant sources). This is especially helpful for endurance athletes, because 3 to 8 percent of energy needs are supplied during endurance exercise by branched-chain amino acids, specifically leucine, isoleucine, and valine. So you definitely need more after exercise to help with muscle repair.

But remember: BCAAs do *not* take the place of whole protein after exercise for muscle protein synthesis. Instead, BCAAs are good for "priming" the brain and muscle to jump-start the mechanistic target of rapamycin, complex-1 (mTORC1) signaling (an essential part of muscle synthesis) once you consume some essential amino acids too.

HYDRATE RIGHT

Paying attention to hydration is always important. It's even more important during the menopausal years, when you may not drink as much as you actually need because you are often not as thirsty as you used to get. This is not to say that you should walk around with a giant jug of plain water to sip on all day. You are likely to just end up peeing most of it out! I see women doing this all the time, and again, it's driven by a commercial culture that pushes jargon-y concepts like "detoxification" and "flushing the system" as a way of selling weight loss and clear skin.

Remember, you have exactly no plain water in your body. All the fluids in your body are a solution that contains electrolytes, glucose, and some amino acids. If you are drinking to hydrate, you want your water to contain small amounts of sugar and salt (not Gatorade levels, mind you!) to activate your transport mechanisms in the gut (technically known as the sodium-glucose co-transport system) and help pull the fluid through your small intestines and into your cells.

Plain water is fine with food, because food provides some sugar and salt going down with the water. But if you are drinking plain water by itself, throughout the day, you can end up peeing out more of what you are consuming and still being just as dehydrated. Instead, mix one teaspoon of maple syrup and ¹⁄₁₆ of a teaspoon of salt into about 10 ounces of water. This gives you 4 grams of carbs from sucrose and 150 milligrams of sodium. This approximately 1 percent solution is perfect for resting and low-intensity hydration.

Chapter 12 will cover hydration *during* exercise.

11

NAIL YOUR NUTRITION TIMING

When you eat is nearly as important as what you eat for optimum performance.

Everyone wants to know what to eat. And there's no question that, as we discussed in the last chapter, the macronutrients and specific foods that you eat are very important for health and performance, especially during your menopausal years. However, another factor that is just as important (if not more so) is often overlooked: *when* you eat.

Nutrient timing is a big part of the equation when you're trying to help your body adapt to the stress of exercise—especially after adding plyometrics and HIIT and LHS—while garnering all the health benefits you can get from combining exercise and good nutrition.

In fact, poor nutrient timing can blunt those benefits, mess with your hormones, disrupt your sleep, and slow your recovery. So don't overlook this final piece of the nutrition puzzle!

EATING AROUND EXERCISE

Everyone focuses on the actual "training" part of training: the gym sessions, the long runs, the hill repeats, and the Masters swim sessions. Those are great. However, you are not getting fitter and faster and stronger *during* those sessions. That's the "damage phase" when you are breaking your body down. And the harder and longer you work, the more you're breaking your body down. You get fitter and faster and stronger *after* those sessions, during the adaptation phase. That's when your body says, "Whoa! What just happened? I need to rally and strengthen the muscles and build the mitochondria and forge some new capillary beds so I'm ready when she wants to do that again!"

How you eat around those sessions—the food you have on board when you start, the food you fuel yourself with during a session, and the food you put in afterward—directly affects how you recover and how you adapt.

As a woman, especially a menopausal woman, you do not want to go into your workouts underfueled. Doing that creates more stress and undermines your exercise progress. You want the macronutrients you need on board to power you through a quality workout so that you're not unduly increasing your stress or eating into your muscle stores. Pre-workout snacks don't have to be complicated, and you don't need to eat a lot. You just want something that contains protein and carbohydrate—a banana with some peanut butter, some dried fruit, granola, a slice of whole grain toast and nut butter—to get the job done.

What you eat afterward is especially important, because your recovery window—the time in which your body is most receptive to restoring your glycogen stores and repairing the muscle damage done—is considerably shorter for you than it is for men. Women need to eat within 30 minutes, whereas men can go up to three hours without eating. That's because we finish hard workouts with high levels of the stress hormone cortisol and in a catabolic state where we are eating into our own muscle stores and breaking down our tissues. As menopausal women, we need to get out of that state as quickly as possible because we can't afford to lose any more muscle and we already are prone to high levels of cortisol, which impedes insulin function.

Eating proper recovery food within 30 minutes of a stressful exercise session pulls your body out of that breakdown state, lowers cortisol, and stimulates your body to start the repair process: pulling carbohydrate back into the liver and muscles and synthesizing that protein into strong, lean muscle tissue. That helps improve your blood sugar control and body composition.

I often see women skipping this important step because they think that not eating after exercise will help them burn more fat. The opposite happens. Their body ends up in a highly stressed state, with high blood sugar, and is more apt to store body fat and slow down metabolism. If you have a recovery snack or meal within that 30-minute window, you can extend your ability to rapidly restore glycogen by up to two hours. It's really important.

Proper recovery nutrition prevents you from getting into a state of low energy availability (LEA), as we talked about in chapter 9, and supports gut microbiome health. Remember, the gut takes a beating during hard exercise. So providing good nutrition when you're done so blood flow is moving from your muscles and back into your gut can help your gut heal and maintain that good bacterial diversity.

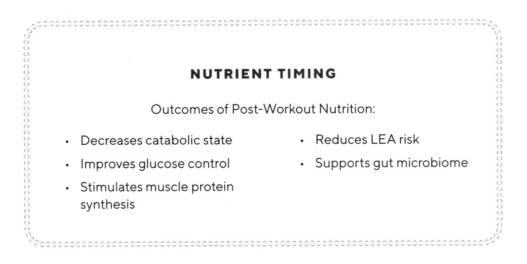

NUTRIENT TIMING

Outcomes of Post-Workout Nutrition:

- Decreases catabolic state
- Improves glucose control
- Stimulates muscle protein synthesis
- Reduces LEA risk
- Supports gut microbiome

Specifically, you want to really focus on protein for recovery. You've probably read that the ideal recovery food or drink has three grams of carbohydrate for every one gram of protein, because protein helps with restocking glycogen and kick-starts muscle repair. That's true. But you also need to be sure you're nailing that 30- to 40-gram mark—specifically, 3 to 3.5 grams of leucine—to really shut down the muscle breakdown process. Then you want to continue to space out your protein throughout the day, getting 30 to 35 grams at each meal so that you maintain that muscle synthesis and a healthy amino acid pool in your circulation.

Animal-based protein like whey tends to be the best source of the essential amino acids (EAAs) that stimulate muscle synthesis. Animal protein is very similar to what our own bodies need for our skeletal muscle. Menopausal women often reach for soy because they want the plant estrogens to relieve menopausal symptoms like hot flashes. The problem is that you need twice as much soy to provide the muscle recovery benefits of animal-based protein like whey. Whey is also an excellent source of leucine. Each 25 grams provides 2.5 grams of leucine. By comparison, you need 40 to 50 grams of soy protein to get the same amount of leucine.

If you're a plant-based athlete and resistant to animal-based proteins, then look for a combination of plant proteins like pea, hemp, and quinoa to get an amino acid profile that is similar to whey.

PROTEIN DOSE, TIMING, AND DISTRIBUTION

MPS = anabolic response that occurs in response to protein feeding and training.	• Specific to leucine intake: ~3 to 3.5g leucine to hit "leucine threshold" in peri- to postmenopausal women.
3-4 meals, evenly spaced, that is >leucine threshold; 0.4g/kg BW (20-40g).	
Best sources: animal protein (particularly whey, egg whites) — due to High BCAA	• Plant based = higher protein intake needed to hit leucine threshold (~50g soy = 25g whey).
MPS "spike" in response to protein feeding, drops back to baseline within 2-3 h.	• Continuous feeding does not help; cell will stop MPS to conserve energy.

Of all the macronutrients, timing and distribution (versus simple total daily intake) are most important for protein.

When you're choosing your protein throughout the day, resist the urge to grab quick fixes. I understand the temptation. Women often feel very rushed and reach for engineered nutrition—protein shakes and bars and drinks—to meet those protein needs throughout the day. And that's okay in a pinch. But don't rely on these products. Shakes, bars, and drinks are classified as highly processed foods, and many of them contain a lot of sugar and other fillers. We always try to avoid and minimize highly processed foods because they are never as good as what nature provides in real foods. They're missing a lot of the vitamins, minerals, and phytonutrients that help your body adapt to stress. You also process the nutrients in real food better than you process engineered foods with added nutrients. For example, when you take a vitamin C tablet, you end up peeing out a lot of the vitamin C. But when you eat an orange, your body absorbs more of it because that food contains the vitamin C along with other nutrients that help your body process it.

It doesn't have to be terribly complicated to eat real food. If you're looking for quick recovery food ideas, you can have a banana with some nut butter or nuts, some fruit and cottage cheese or a handful of nuts, Greek yogurt and low-sugar granola, whole wheat crackers and some tuna, or some veggies and quinoa. Again, in a pinch, a high-quality protein drink is okay. But save it for when you need it.

There are also plenty of protein-rich post-workout meals that are easy to grab and go. Try avocado and eggs on toast; salmon and brown rice; grilled chicken salad, or a veggie and hummus pita. Once you have a set repertoire of recovery snacks and meals, it becomes easier and easier to eat what you need to without relying on ready-made, highly processed foods.

Snack and meal ideas for before or after a workout:

Smoothie	Vegetables with quinoa
Salmon and brown rice	Dried fruit
Banana with peanut butter	Boiled eggs
Whole grain toast and eggs	Grilled chicken salad
Cottage cheese	Whole wheat crackers and tuna
Granola bar	Chicken and vegetables
Greek yogurt with granola	Nuts

KACIE,* 56, is an avid Olympic and power lifter. She started having menopause symptoms at 51, and is now postmenopausal. She feels that she has lost a significant amount of muscle, becoming "squishy" overnight, and is no longer making progress in her lifts. Her goal: Get those muscles back.

GENERAL ASSESSMENT

Kacie is 5'5", 148 pounds, and 25 percent body fat. So she's in a healthy range, but has been experiencing a significant drop in lean muscle mass and an increase in body fat. Because of the body composition changes she's experiencing, she's wondering if she should try the estradiol patch to help with muscle mass.

She is really into power lifting and Olympic lifting and does a bit of CrossFit for HIIT training. She does most of her CrossFit sessions fasted in the early morning and then does her Olympic lifting sessions in the afternoon. The first step is to stop all this fasted training, because it's not good anytime of the day. The double-sessions, especially with the morning fasted CrossFit was also creating too much stress, too much cortisol, and not enough recovery time, which was perpetuating the fat gain and muscle loss.

If she wanted to keep her early morning CrossFit, then she needed to eat something before and have breakfast after. We also needed to modulate some of her intensity. If she wants to do the CrossFit, then she needs to scale it to complement her evening session in the gym, so she's not doing all top-end intensity all the time.

Nutritionally, she tries to stay away from processed foods, but does rely pretty heavily on protein powder, which she has with her all the time. We want to broaden her nutrition and include more foods that are nutrient dense to support a healthy gut microbiome. I also had her start using ashwagandha and schisandra to bring down cortisol and help her be more stress resilient without reaching for an estrogen patch, which won't help with developing muscle mass.

HER NEW ROUTINE

Here's how her new schedule looks after our makeover:

MONDAY: 6 to 7 a.m. CrossFit. She has a lot of friends in that class, so we keep that in the schedule, but her goal is to maintain a rating of perceived exertion (RPE) between 5 and 6 on a 1 to 10 scale, not to go all out and not to worry about hitting all the prescribed intensities of that class; it is just about moving the body and being a bit social. She's no longer doing it fasted, and instead eats before and immediately after, with each mini meal containing 20 grams of protein. We keep the 7 p.m. yoga, but bring it out of the studio and have her do it at home so she can really relax and focus, and not fight traffic on the way home, which helps her maintain that parasympathetic (rest and digest) activity.

TUESDAY: 6 to 7 a.m. CrossFit, eating before and immediately after as before. Again, she's to maintain an RPE of 5, knowing that her true focus of the day is hitting her hard lifts that evening at 6 p.m. at her Olympic Lifting Club.

WEDNESDAY: Sleep in. No CrossFit. This lets her be her freshest and have focus for her 6 p.m. Olympic Lifting Club.

THURSDAY: Busy work day and a two hour technique session with her coach that evening. She has a little coffee and schisandra in the afternoon before that session to give her a boost and mental lift. She packs a baggie of nuts and dates to snack on during the session, along with some BCAAs in her hydration drink. She notices the benefits of this immediately with better reaction time and lifting focus.

FRIDAY: 8 to 9:30 CrossFit with extra mobility. This is a little later in the morning so she can sleep in. It is also a more moderate-intensity class that focuses on mobility work instead of that high intensity. She has coffee and breakfast with friends afterward.

SATURDAY: 8 to 10:30 a.m. Olympic Lifting session with a focus on competition. So this is where she wants to be her freshest to work on her weaknesses and focus on specific lifts for upcoming competitions.

SUNDAY: Off or play day at the gym, working on mobility and catching up socially. The goal is to have fun and relax.

She has also periodized her training so every week is not the same. She'll have two weeks on where the training is hard and heavy and one week of "de-load," where she takes the weight down and focuses on technique and recovery.

FUELING DURING EXERCISE

You've undoubtedly heard all the carbohydrate recommendations for exercise, with some suggesting that you take in up to 80 or 90 grams per hour! It won't surprise you that a lot of those recommendations are based on the energy needs of young men, but frankly, I don't typically recommend specific carbohydrate grams per hour for either men or women. Why? Because there are sex differences in how we feel during exercise: Men use more carbohydrate, tapping into their liver and muscle stores; but women clear their blood sugar and use fat rather than fully deplete their liver and muscle glycogen. Women especially benefit from taking in calories from whole foods, which contain a blend of protein, carbs, and fat, to fuel their exercise. They're less likely to feel bloated and gassy and uncomfortably full during long efforts with mixed macronutrients than they will if they keep trying to shovel down more carbs than their gut can process.

I'll note that, for menopausal women, energy products that contain a lot of fructose (fruit sugar) are particularly problematic, because we have an even harder time metabolizing fructose than women still in their reproductive years. Research dating back to the 1960s shows that postmenopausal women end up with more fatty acids in their blood after drinking fructose-laden beverages than they do if they consume glucose-based drinks. Postmenopausal women also can't store excess energy from fructose as well as premenopausal women can. While premenopausal women can store excess energy from fructose in their subcutaneous fat stores (hips and thighs), postmenopausal women are not able to do so and end up with more fatty acids circulating in their bloodstream, where it causes high triglyceride levels and insulin resistance. As a consequence, if you're trying to fuel with fructose-heavy products, you're not getting the energy you need and you're also risking "gut rot": the cramping, bloating, and nausea you feel when your carbohydrates are just sitting in your gut. Eating mixed macronutrient real food solves this issue.

A good fueling range for active women is 0.9 to 1.13 calories per pound of body weight (so, 140 calories an hour for a 140-pound woman) per hour of running (or a similar activity that mechanically jostles the gut) and 1.3 to 1.6 calories per pound (so, 225 calories for that same woman) while cycling or engaging in another non-jostling activity. When in doubt, err toward the lesser amount. It helps avoid that gut rot from eating more than your already taxed stomach can handle.

A word here about gels. Anyone who has followed me for any amount of time knows that I do not recommend standard carbohydrate gels during exercise. One standard gel packet ranges from 100 to 120 calories per serving—typically about 25 to 30 grams of carbs—and is made up of maltodextrin and fructose with a bit of sodium, potassium, flavorings, and preservatives. You'll see on the label of most gel products that the gel must be consumed with two to four ounces of water. That's because a gel is very concentrated carbohydrate. If you don't consume it with an adequate amount of water, it cannot get out of your stomach and into your gut where it can be absorbed for energy. Without enough water, your body has to pull from its own fluid reserve to water down that gel so you can use it, effectively dehydrating you. Gels also contain a blend of carbohydrates that can overload the transport receptors in your gut, forcing your body, once again, to pull in some fluid to dilute what is sitting in there. You end up with "goo gut": bloating, gas, diarrhea, nausea, and general GI discomfort. For the best results, stick to real food.

HOW TO HYDRATE

You can't necessarily trust your thirst right now.

I've been studying hydration from one angle or another my entire adult life (the basis of my PhD was sex differences in hydration in the heat!), both as an athlete myself in endurance running, Ironman triathlon, pro-elite road cycling, and CrossFit and as a nutrition and physiology researcher working in the lab as well as the field with elite professional athletes. There is absolutely no question in my mind that hydration is power.

Very often athletes will think they need to eat more when they find themselves tiring, but in fact what they really need to do is hydrate more . . . and hydrate properly. That last part is key. Though our understanding of hydration has definitely evolved, the bestselling hydration drink on the market is still the one that was created on a football field 40 years ago, and it still has more carbs and calories than are needed for hydration, especially for women. Many of these mainstream commercial drinks not only are poorly optimized for hydration but can impair performance by creating GI distress and, effectively, dehydration, because they're poorly absorbed and an athlete's body has to pull fluid out of the blood and muscles to dilute them.

The goal of this book is to deliver physiology, training, and nutrition advice that is specific to women in their menopause transition, so I haven't covered much of the basic ground that I did in *ROAR*. I'm making an exception for this chapter, because the nuts and bolts of hydration are very important. (I also don't want to assume that you've read *ROAR* or make you buy it to get that information if you have not.) So the following is a refresher on hydration from *ROAR*, revised to address your specific needs at this part of your active journey.

HYDRATION 101: THE QUEST TO KEEP YOU COOL

The main point of hydration is to keep your body fluid levels high enough to continue functioning properly. You use the water in your body to get rid of the heat you produce and to cool you down while you're exercising. When everything is working properly, it's an amazingly efficient process. Your blood circulates to your muscles to deliver fuel and nutrients, as well as to sweep up the waste and heat that your muscles produce while they're working. The blood then circulates to your skin to dump the heat through evaporative cooling (sweating).

Sweat works by pulling water (which comes from the plasma) from your blood through your skin, where it can evaporate and cool you down. The more you sweat, the more your blood plasma volume drops. So your body needs to pull water from other spaces to keep your blood volume high enough to continue sweating. If you slack on your hydration, you won't have enough fluid in your body to keep your blood volume high enough to sweat efficiently and cool yourself. With less water in your blood, the blood is more viscous, so your heart has to work harder. Your heart rate goes up. Your power goes down. Your core temperature rises. All of that leads to fatigue, reduced performance, and the dreaded power decline at the end of a hard workout.

This whole scenario sets up a serious competition between your muscles and your skin. As soon as you start to exercise, your muscles and your skin fight over your blood, one to keep your muscles pumping and the other to keep your body cool. As the level of your body water drops, this competition becomes fiercer. Ultimately, your muscles win this round (though as you'll see in a second, they don't really win the fight): less blood goes to the skin so that more fuel can reach your working muscles. With less blood going to the skin, there's less sweat to keep you cool and your risk for heat illness goes up.

Obviously, this situation can't continue indefinitely. Eventually, your working muscles and your cooling system will both need more blood than your cardiovascular system can supply. When your body reaches this point, you can't keep your temperature in check, and these temperature points usually signal the body to stop exercise. The first aspect of fatigue is the tipping point of a muscle temperature over 102 degrees Fahrenheit; at that point the contractile proteins start to break down. The second point is a core temperature reaching 104 to 105.8 degrees Fahrenheit (40 to 41 degrees Celsius); a core temperature this high signals changes to the central nervous system to slow down or stop exercise. Note here that it's not just core temperature that hinders your performance, but the overall heat stress you're experiencing and your limited blood circulation.

This perfect storm of hot skin, low body water, and high core temperature makes it impossible for your muscles to perform the job at hand, whether it's pedaling, running, rowing, or whatever you want them to do.

You assume that drinking fluids will fix this problem, but that is not always the case. As I mentioned before, often it's **what** you're drinking that's making you dehydrated. The mass hydration market out there has saturated the general public with the message that when you drink a 5 to 8 percent carbohydrate solution with sodium (roughly 12 to 19 grams of carbohydrate with 52 to 110 milligrams of sodium per 8 ounces), you are taking care of your hydration, sodium, and fueling needs. The focus is always on carbohydrate availability and calories. I've done extensive research and have been dismayed to find that the focus of hydration research is far too often on carbs as liquid calories. As a physiologist who specializes in hydration, thermoregulation, and performance, I find this to be a misleading and incorrect message.

PUMP UP THE VOLUME

Now that you understand the basics of hydration, let's take a look at how fluid gets from your bottle and into your bloodstream. It starts in your gut, specifically your small intestines, where 95 percent of all fluid absorption happens. The small intestines are very sensitive to water and sodium and act like Lady Justice in the body, trying to keep the two in balance so that your blood plasma has just the right level of osmolality. Normal blood plasma osmolality is between 275 and 295 milliosmoles. I don't expect you to remember that, but it will help you understand how hydration works.

For the fluid you're pouring down your throat and into your belly to make its way into your bloodstream swiftly and efficiently, you should make sure it's a fluid of lower osmolality than your blood (ideally between 210 and 260 milliosmoles). Why? Basic science. If your blood is more concentrated than the fluid you drink, your small intestinal cells will let that fluid through the intestinal walls to add water to the bloodstream and lower the concentration levels.

On the flip side, if you take in fluid that is too concentrated, your intestinal cells will reverse course and pull water from the vascular spaces of your body to dilute the higher osmolality in your gut. In other words, water leaves the spaces where you want it and goes into your digestive system to dilute the fluid sitting in your gut. As you might imagine, the last thing you want is to have water pouring into the small intestines when you're trying to hydrate. In the end, you may have effectively dehydrated yourself and triggered GI distress to boot.

The composition (as well as the concentration) of the fluid you're drinking is also important. For optimum hydration, your body relies on what are called fluid co-transporters, which are essentially molecular pilots that carry fluid across your intestinal cells and into the water spaces of the body.

Sodium, a *Top Gun*–level pilot for hydration, works best when it has a good co-pilot—and glucose is the co-pilot of choice. Sodium is absorbed into your cells by a few mechanisms, but mostly it hitches a ride with glucose. Without glucose, the constant flow of sodium and water into your bloodstream slows down. This is why sports drinks that actually hydrate (instead of sitting in the stomach, causing sloshing, bloat, and discomfort) contain a small amount of sugar (glucose and sucrose) as well as sodium for optimal absorption and hydration.

This is also why plain water isn't optimal for hydration. Water contains no drivers, and like a fluid that is too concentrated, it may just slosh around for a while before it gets where it needs to go. Plain water also can cause a volume response—signaling your body to pee out more than you've taken in.

THE WINNING (AND NOT WINNING) SOLUTION

So what's the winning solution for hydration? Not the "solution" that so many recreational (and even professional) athletes use. Here are the nutritional aspects of a typical carb-heavy sports drink:

- *5 to 8 percent carbohydrate solution (12 to 19 grams of carbs per 8 ounces)*
- *Osmolality of around 300 to 305 milliosmoles*
- *Sugars: maltodextrin, fructose, sucrose*
- *Sodium: 52 to 110 milligrams per 8 ounces*

That sports drink does, of course, provide some carbohydrates, but not at the levels you need to sustain long-term endurance exercise. Sports drinks often contain maltodextrin and fructose, which are notorious for causing GI distress. Instead, you want to seek out a sports drink that supplies some glucose, sodium, and other key co-transporters, as described earlier. A winning solution contains:

- *3 to 4 percent carbohydrate solution (3 to 4 grams of carbs per 100 milliliters [3.38 oz], or 7 to 9.4 grams per 8 ounces)*

- *Sugars: 7 to 9.4 grams from glucose and sucrose*
- *Sodium: 180 to 225 milligrams*
- *Potassium (another fluid co-transporter that can help sodium): 60 to 75 milligrams*

SALTY SWEATERS AND SHAKERS

It's true that sodium is important for healthy hydration, but unfortunately, a lot of athletes get stuck on the issue of salt. I counsel a lot of Kona-bound triathletes, and nearly all of them will ask if they need to take salt tablets or take sodium-based electrolyte supplements. Their concern is understandable. Hawaii is hot, you sweat a lot when it's hot, and you lose a lot of sodium when you sweat a lot, especially if you're a salty sweater. (That's you with the white streaks on your helmet straps, running cap, or face.)

The short answer is an emphatic no—you do not need salt tablets! Even as a salty sweater, your body has ample sodium stores, and you will consume plenty of sodium from the foods you are eating and drinking (if you choose your hydration source wisely). You're taking in sodium to work with your physiology under exercise stress conditions, not trying to replace sodium. In the human body, fluid is made up of water and electrolytes, and the key electrolyte that allows fluid to move freely is sodium.

Salt tablets stress the GI system more than most people realize. The chloride ion of sodium chloride (common salt), which is necessary for cellular function, is lost through sweat, but not at rates high enough to warrant dumping in high loads during exercise. The chloride ion interferes with what we call the membrane potential of the intestinal cells; it allows the spaces between the cells to open up and release gut bacteria, which, in turn, causes an abnormal water flux and severe diarrhea. Furthermore, when you ingest a high dose of sodium, you end up with a bit of reverse water flux. If you have a high concentration of sodium in the digestive tract, water will leach into your GI tract to try to dilute the salt rather than be absorbed into the blood. This contributes to dehydration and that awful feeling of gut sloshing.

In a nutshell: you don't need salt tablets, and taking them can actually impair your performance. What you do need is a physiologically sound sports drink that supplies around 360 to 450 milligrams of sodium per 16 ounces. The typical diet has plenty of added sodium, but if you eat a very minimally processed diet, go ahead and be more liberal with your salt shaker. You can also eat more sodium-rich foods like anchovies, smoked salmon, pickles, and salted nuts to keep yourself well hydrated, especially when you're exercising a lot in the heat.

DRINK ACCORDING TO THIRST? USE SENSE INSTEAD!

For far too many years, endurance athletes—especially those who were exercising for many hours, like marathoners, Ironman triathletes, and long-distance cyclists—were urged to prevent dehydration by drinking early, often, and before they were thirsty, the idea being that more was better. That practice had some grave consequences in the form of hyponatremia, or dangerously low blood sodium. In fact, one study conducted on participants in the 2002 Boston marathon found that 13 percent finished with hyponatremia, and the majority of them were women. Selene did a podcast with Duke University yoga therapist Carol Krucoff, who ended up in a coma for four days as a result of severe hyponatremia after running a marathon in Jamaica.

So yes, you can drink too much, and hyponatremia is a real risk. Reflexively, trainers and coaches started advising athletes to drink according to thirst. Period. No more. No less. This is okay as a very general starting point, but if you take the message too far, you can end up not drinking enough. Sometimes thirst is not an accurate indicator of your hydration level.

There are a few issues with drinking according to thirst, and one is that the basic research behind the recommendation has been done on men. There is a significant sex difference (and age difference for that matter) when it comes to thirst sensation. Let's go back to those two key female hormones, estrogen and progesterone. Both affect your hypothalamus—the part of the brain that regulates fatigue as well as fluid balance hormones. When these hormones are high, estrogen lowers the threshold for feeling thirsty and lowers the trigger point for vasopressin release. (That release happens through an anti-diuretic hormone, or ADH, which forms in the hypothalamus. ADH prevents the loss of water from your body by reducing the amount you pee and helping the kidneys reabsorb water into your body.) At the same time, progesterone is converted to cortisol and attaches to the same receptor site as aldosterone, which signals the body to kick out additional sodium.

This change alone makes you, as a woman, more predisposed to hyponatremia. High hormone levels reset your body's signals to respond to a lower plasma volume (up to 8 percent lower). That simply means that your drive to drink or your level of thirst, which is driven by plasma osmolality and volume, is dampened. So even if your body is dehydrated, you may not feel thirsty. This can become more pronounced during perimenopause as your hormones start to fluctuate, sometimes dramatically.

Similarly, have you ever done a tough workout on a warm or hot day and when you get home you feel a bit sick, but not all that thirsty? Physiologically, you are dehydrated, but systemic dehydration has kicked in to lessen your desire for water and food. In this instance, your body is telling you not to drink, even though that is what you actually need. And the most important thing to remember is that your body's normal reaction to exercise is an increase in blood sodium levels, not a decrease, as you lose more water from your blood via sweat; thus, your blood becomes more "concentrated" with solutes like sodium.

Lack of thirst only gets worse as we get older, especially for postmenopausal women who have low levels of thirst. One study compared the sweat rate, sweat volume, sweat sodium content, and level of thirst among three groups of women—premenopausal (average age 22), perimenopausal (average age 46), and postmenopausal (average age 52) as they exercised on a treadmill. The perimenopausal women had the highest sweat rates (which the authors attributed to the disruption of thermoregulation that leads to hot flashes and night sweats during this time), and the postmenopausal women had the lowest levels of thirst, which makes sense, since they weren't sweating as much. However, the postmenopausal women were also more likely to be cooking inside, so ideally they should have started sweating earlier and getting the cues to drink sooner.

Thirst is generally not reliable for you right now. An exception may be if you are taking menopausal hormone therapy (MHT). Research finds that estrogen therapy increases osmotic sensitivity for mechanisms to retain body water, so it may help menopausal women regulate their fluid levels and avoid dehydration.

So how much should you drink? You can start by drinking to thirst, but also use common sense. We're far better off using sex-specific guidelines to reduce the risk of heat illness as well as hyponatremia. Everyone is an individual, so your fluid needs may be very different from those of your teammate or training partner. The old recommendation was to drink to replace body weight loss during exercise (you have probably heard the advice to weigh yourself before and after exercise to determine how many ounces you lost), but doing so can contribute to overdrinking and does not account for body weight loss from fuel burned (glycogen) or any residual fluid or food left in your gut that you consumed during exercise.

Generally speaking, taking in fluids at the rate of 0.12 ounces per pound of body weight (that's about 17 ounces for a 140-pound woman) per hour in temperatures 75 degrees Fahrenheit and below, and 0.16 ounces per pound of body weight (roughly 22 ounces for the same woman) per hour in temperatures about 80 degrees Fahrenheit will maintain blood volume and delay muscle fatigue. Smaller women may need less and larger women may need more. Use the guidelines that follow to determine whether you should drink to thirst or if you are better off following a hydration schedule.

DRINK TO THIRST DURING EXERCISE IF:

- *You have prehydrated prior to the training session or race. (If you have not, dehydration can predispose you to tissue injury, decreased motivation during exercise, and poor recovery.)*

- *You are heat-acclimated.*

- *You are adequately trained. (After significant time off resulting in lower fitness levels, dehydration and exercise stress can exacerbate thermal strain and decrease your performance metrics.)*

- *You are on MHT.*

- *You have a history of exercise-associated hyponatremia (EAH) or have SIADH (syndrome of inappropriate antidiuretic hormone) secretion.*

DRINK ON A SCHEDULE DURING EXERCISE IF:

- *You have two or more heavy training sessions in a day (to avoid systemic dehydration).*

- *You are not acclimated to heat and/or altitude and are training in these conditions.*

- *You have a history of heat illness.*

EVERYONE CAN HYPERHYDRATE

I'm a big proponent of prehydrating. Starting the night before a big event, especially if you're in the high hormone phase or if you're postmenopausal and have noticed your thirst isn't kicking in like it used to, you can hyperhydrate by drinking sodium-rich fluids like chicken broth or miso soup. There are non-sports-related products that work well as a hyperhydration drink, such as Ural (a urinary alkalinizer used for cystitis and urinary tract infections that is high in sodium), and sport nutrition products that are sodium-based hyperhydration mixes.

Prehydrating is one of the single most effective strategies I've used with endurance athletes like Selene, who tells me that she feels like she has bonus watts on her bike when she starts a race or a ride with a bottle of preload in her system. As she told me, "It's extremely helpful, especially now that I'm postmenopausal and I find heat harder to handle."

LIGHT SPORTS DRINKS: BUYER BEWARE

As more and more athletes are concerned about consuming too many carbs, some sports drinks now offer "lighter" low-calorie mixes. But buyer beware. For starters, these drinks do nothing to shepherd fluid through the intestinal wall. A bit of glucose and sodium is needed to work with the physiology of the small intestines and pull fluid in (remember the glucose-sodium co-transport system).

Some of these products contain sugar substitutes, which you absolutely don't want. Certain types of sugar substitutes, particularly sugar alcohols like sorbitol, mannitol, and xylitol, pull water into the GI tract and out of the blood. These ingredients are more commonly used as laxatives and strongly linked to GI distress—that's the opposite of what you're looking for! The natural sweetener Stevia is currently popular. Some athletes tolerate it, but many women find it bitter and can experience bloating and other GI issues from using it.

Other sugar substitutes can cause your blood sugar to crash. For example, when you consume sucralose, your body perceives the sweetness and releases insulin in anticipation of the sugar to come. But there is no sugar, and so your existing blood glucose gets taken up—causing a drop in blood glucose and a bit of hypoglycemia. This signals your body to release more glucose into the blood, which, in turn, causes more insulin to be released, and around and around it goes. During exercise, insulin doesn't play a large role in blood sugar control, but ingesting products with sucralose can make your blood sugar bottom out more quickly (kind of like taking in lots of caffeine), thus increasing your need for carbohydrates. Recent studies have also found that chronic consumption of sucralose may lead to greater insulin resistance.

13

SLEEP WELL AND RECOVER RIGHT

How to get the rest and regeneration you need to stay fit and fresh.

There's a reason why professional athletes like golfer Michelle Wie swear by sleep. And I mean *lots* of sleep: according to *Golf Digest,* Wie claims to have once slept 16 hours straight and aims for 10 hours of shuteye a night (or did pre-baby!) to stay on top of her game.

It's the same reason why trainer Erin Carson, based in Boulder, Colorado, has found success in training superstar athletes like three-time Ironman World Champion Mirinda Carfrae and success as a triathlete herself, qualifying for Ironman 70.3—Nice when she was 53 and finishing 25th in her age group in Worlds 70.3 at age 54. Erin is vigilant about sleep and usually drifts off by 8 p.m. so that she can be fresh and ready for her 4:30 a.m. wake-up call.

Though there are certainly other techniques that are helpful for repair and performance, sleep and recovery are inextricably connected.

Unfortunately, menopause and midlife can send dueling wrecking balls straight into your sleep architecture, leaving you tossing and turning and unable to get to sleep, waking up with racing thoughts at 3 a.m., and generally feeling unable to get the rest and regeneration you need. So before we get to the other recovery pieces, let's first tackle sleep.

HOW SLEEP WORKS

Deep sleep is when you produce the majority of one of your body's greatest performance enhancers, human growth hormone (HGH), which helps you burn fat and stimulates tissue growth to build muscle and allow you to recover faster. When you shortchange your sleep—getting fewer than seven to nine hours a night—your HGH production stalls. That slump is particularly pronounced when you go to bed late, says renowned sleep specialist W. Christopher Winter, author of *The Sleep Solution: Why Your Sleep Is Broken and How to Fix It.*

"The majority of your body's HGH secretion happens between 11 p.m. and 1 a.m. and then it starts shutting down," says Winter. Your production of HGH also naturally declines with age. Estrogen helps increase HGH during our premenopausal years. It declines as our estrogen declines, so it's important to try to get to bed earlier and take advantage of that HGH production window, especially during your menopausal years.

Inadequate sleep is also stressful on your body. The levels of stress hormones like cortisol, which menopausal women already struggle to keep in check, remain elevated deep into the evening hours when they would naturally begin to decline. Research shows that cortisol declines six times more slowly in people who are short on sleep than in those who are properly rested. That not only messes with your moods but wrecks your recovery by impairing tissue repair and growth. It also sets the stage for insulin resistance, increased abdominal fat storage (which menopausal women do not need), injury, and overtraining.

You're more prone to overeating when you're tired. Research indicates that sleep deprivation is linked to higher levels of the appetite stimulator ghrelin and lower levels of the appetite suppressor leptin. That's why you might find yourself constantly grazing or on the hunt for sugary snacks after a night (or more) of short sleep.

It's also hard for your body to restock your glycogen stores when you don't get enough sleep. Prolonged sleep deprivation blunts insulin response. Research suggests even one night of sleep deprivation can reduce insulin sensitivity by 33 percent. That in turn impairs your body's ability to restock its glycogen supply, which you need to feel fresh and fully recovered.

And it's not just your muscles that suffer. Hard training like sprint workouts and CrossFit sessions demand lots of ATP (adenosine triphosphate) to power you through. The by-product of burning through ATP is adenosine, which builds up in your brain (making you drowsy) as well as in your body. "The only way to clear it out is sleep," says Winter. Once you slip into slumber, your brain fires up the cleanup crews and clears the adenosine, which makes room for your brain to restock its own glycogen supply. Without sleep, the waste products remain and your brain doesn't get all the energy it needs.

Of course, you don't perform at your best when you're not properly rested. Your reaction time slows down and your endurance performance suffers when you don't get enough sleep. Exercise also feels harder. Research shows that how rested you are impacts your perceived exertion during exercise. So when you're fully rested, those hard sessions feel relatively easy; when you're not rested, they very much don't.

This does not mean that your marathon or big event you've been training months for will be wrecked if you spend the night before tossing and turning with nervous energy. Multiple studies have shown that one night of disrupted sleep, especially before an event, doesn't hurt endurance or power. Your race day energy will be fine. It's chronically poor sleep we're concerned about.

SLEEP AND RECOVERY TRACKING

If you tune into yourself, you can generally tell when you're well rested and recovered. You have a spring in your step and you can bound up the stairs without feeling like you're scaling Everest.

Modern technology also can help. Devices like the Whoop Strap and the Oura Ring monitor your activity during the day and track your heart rate, respiration rate, body temperature, and sleep stages. They also monitor many other sleep metrics at night, like restfulness, latency (how long it takes you to fall asleep), and sleep efficiency, deliver sleep and readiness scores, and give you activity recommendations based on those scores.

These devices work remarkably well and allow you to clearly see the consequences of your behavior (both good and bad). Too much wine before bed? You can see your recovery and readiness drop as your heart rate stays elevated later into the night and you fail to drift into the deeper, restorative sleep stages you need. Early to bed with a book? You can see your recovery rise.

That's the real benefit of these devices: they allow you to peer into your own physiology. So, as you're trying adaptogens, new training techniques, dietary shifts, and lifestyle interventions, you can see what is or isn't working and adjust accordingly. They also help you stay on track. No one likes getting a low score, so knowing that staying up to watch just one more episode of your favorite Netflix binge or topping off that glass of wine before bed will dock you some rest and readiness points (not to mention actually harm your health and performance in real life), you're more likely to do what you know you should do.

These devices should not be taken as gospel, however, for what kind of day you're going to have, especially when it comes to recovery. Their recovery scores are based on cardiovascular strain, not total body strain. So your legs may feel like they're full of wet cement from a hard weight session, but you wake up with a bright green ready-to-go score on your tracking app, even though you are most certainly not ready to go for more than an active recovery day.

THE MENOPAUSE SLEEP CONUNDRUM

Not surprisingly, when women come to me saying that they're having a hard time coming around in their training and never feel fresh, sleep is one of the first things we look at, given its role in performance and recovery. Disrupted sleep is especially likely to be the culprit if they're in their menopausal years, because those hormonal fluctuations can wreak havoc on sleep.

Progesterone helps control stress, lets you relax and chill, and has a direct sedative effect. As levels drop during menopause, it's harder to fall and stay asleep. Estrogen increases REM (deep dream) sleep, assists serotonin metabolism (so you can relax), and may decrease sleep latency (how long it takes you to fall asleep). Estrogen also decreases the number of times you wake in the night, increases total sleep time and quality, and helps regulate the stress hormone cortisol to stabilize sleep. It helps regulate your internal thermostat and body temperature, which is essential for restful sleep. The decline in estrogen levels can lead to hot flashes and disruptive night sweats and make you more susceptible to nighttime cortisol spikes, even from mild stress like ambient noise and light. Women also start producing less melatonin, which is a key hormone for regulating sleep and helping the body cool down enough to trigger optimal sleep.

Unsurprisingly, given all this, about 61 percent of postmenopausal women struggle with some amount of insomnia, according to the Sleep Foundation. A 2017 study published by the Centers for Disease Control and Prevention paints a more complete—and unfortunately similar—picture.

Among women ages 40 to 59, the CDC study found that perimenopausal women in that age range reported being the least likely to get at least seven hours of sleep. About 40 percent of postmenopausal women in the study said that they slept less than seven hours a night, compared to 56 percent of perimenopausal women and 32.5 percent of premenopausal women.

Postmenopausal women in the report were more likely than premenopausal women of the same age to have trouble falling asleep (27.1 percent compared with 16.8 percent), and to have trouble staying asleep (35.9 percent compared with 23.7 percent) four times or more a week.

Postmenopausal women in this age range were also more likely (55 percent) than their premenopausal counterparts (47 percent) to not wake up feeling rested most days of the week.

So now you know: you're really not alone. And the last thing I want to do is cause you even more stress about lack of sleep and heighten your anxiety while you're lying in bed with racing thoughts, trying to will yourself to relax and rest.

So what to do? Sleep is essential enough to warrant a multipronged approach to reclaiming it and all of its recovery and health benefits. So we'll start with basic sleep hygiene advice and then get specific about how to manage the challenges presented by menopause.

HEALTHY SLEEP PRACTICES

When sleep is elusive, you need to take a few more steps to pave the way for it, especially during the menopausal years, when fluctuating hormones conspire to keep you awake.

Ideally, you want to set the stage for your body to cycle through all four stages of quality sleep; characterized by different brain activity, the four stages make up what sleep experts call your sleep architecture:

> *Stage 1: Brain drifting out of conscious thought and into sleep*
>
> *Stage 2: Light sleep*
>
> *Stage 3: Deep, restorative sleep*
>
> *Stage 4: REM sleep, where your muscle tone goes limp and you enter dream sleep*

To help maintain a healthy sleep architecture:

CORK THE BOTTLE BEFORE BEDTIME: Many women (and men, but this book is for women) use alcohol to wind down at the end of the day or have a nightcap to help feel drowsy so they can drift off to sleep. And it works . . . temporarily. A glass or two of Shiraz may leave you nodding off during your favorite Netflix series. But it ultimately lessens the quality of your sleep and increases restlessness toward the early morning hours, especially if you're drinking right before bed.

Drinking within an hour of bedtime lengthens your non-REM sleep and shortens your REM sleep during the first half of the night; as a result, you don't get into that deep restorative sleep for very long. As your liver sops up the ethanol from your bloodstream, your body can go into a bit of withdrawal during the second half of the night, making you restless and more likely to toss and turn. Avoiding alcohol can also help reduce the number and severity of hot flashes. So have that glass with dinner, but switch over to tart cherry juice (more on that in a bit) before bedtime. Your sleep will thank you.

MOVE UP DINNERTIME: Making your body work on digestion can interfere with your parasympathetic needs during sleep. This is especially true if you have a larger meal, which can cause indigestion that you may not even register, but that wakes you up enough to be disruptive and prevents you from falling into those deep, restorative sleep stages. Give yourself at least two hours, preferably three, before your last meal and bedtime.

Now, I know what you're thinking, because I hear it often. "But I have a swim workout (track session, bike race) in the evening, and I don't get home until eight, and I want to be in bed by ten. How do I manage that?" That schedule does make it difficult to not eat within two hours of bedtime. So I generally recommend that athletes work backwards: Have a light dinner around 4:00 or 4:30 and your race or workout session at 5:30 or 6:00. Then have a protein-rich snack directly afterward. By the time you wind down to be in bed, you won't have a bellyful of food. Alternatively, if you regularly exercise in the evening and get home late every night, you could make your main meal a really large lunch in the early afternoon, then have a mini-meal before and after training.

TURN OFF THE SCREENS: You've heard it before: shut down the electronics—including your phone—30 minutes before you want to be sleeping. Do you do it? Most of us don't. If sleep eludes you, it is very much worth practicing this bedtime ritual. When you're lying there with your phone, tablet, or laptop, you're bathing your eyes in blue light, which has been shown to suppress the production of melatonin, and your melatonin is already dwindling with age. Your body temperature won't fall as it should (which, again, is really important for menopausal women), and you won't get the signal that it's time for sleep. Yes, you can buy blue light–blocking computer glasses. But really, the best way to wind down is with a soft reading light and a book.

KEEP YOUR COOL: The best temperature for a solid night of shuteye is about 65 degrees, give or take, depending on your preference. That's especially important for menopausal women who are prone to hot flashes and night sweats. You can also keep cool by switching to cooling pajamas made from naturally wicking fibers like bamboo. (Many companies now make PJs designed to keep menopausal women comfortable.) You wear performance clothes when you work out. Why not wear performance PJs for optimum recovery? You can find cooling sheets, mattress toppers, and even mattresses that will help keep you in the comfortable sleep temperature zone.

I also recommend taking a cool shower before bedtime to help bring down your core temperature and lull you to sleep as well. Start with the water on warm (so you don't shock your system) and gradually turn the hot water down until the temperature is cool and you feel chilled. Then get in your PJs, curl up in your sheets, and feel the pleasant tiredness wash over you.

BLOCK OUT THE STIMULATION: Ambient light and noise can keep you from drifting into that deep restorative state of sleep. Hang some blackout curtains and turn on a white noise machine to block out the sleep disturbing light and sound, both of which you may be especially sensitive to at this time of life. Or simply try wearing a sleep mask and earplugs if you find them comfortable enough.

KEEP A BEDSIDE PAD AND PEN: If you have a busy mind at bedtime, those galloping active beta brain waves will leave you skimming the surface of sleep without allowing you to drift into the deep, slower brain wave stages. To satisfy your inner problem-solver, write down what's occupying your mind before you go to bed, including the steps you'll take the next day to address them. If you wake up in the night with more thoughts that won't let you rest, grab that pen and pad and jot them down instead of lying there letting them race around inside your head. It will help you get back to sleep.

FLIP YOUR EXERCISE TIME: Contrary to what you may have heard, exercising in the evening is not an automatic sleep-wrecker. In fact, it can be better than dragging yourself out of bed at 5 a.m. after a restless night and then sleepwalking through the day. A 2019 meta-analysis of 23 studies found that evening exercise not only had no negative effect on sleep but also sometimes improved it, as long as the session wrapped up at least an hour before bedtime. For an even better sleep-inducer, top off your sweat session with a cool shower to bring your body temperature down and set the stage for quality shuteye.

GO EASY ON THE ESPRESSO: What's the first thing you do when you're dragging during the day? If you're like many women, you reach for another (and another) cup of coffee. But that can set you up for a vicious cycle as too much caffeine wrecks your sleep and leaves you dragging into another day. Remember that chemical called adenosine that clears during sleep? Even without hard exercise, it builds during the day and binds to specific nerve receptors to make you feel drowsy. Caffeine is an adenosine decoy that floats through your bloodstream and binds to those receptors. So now, instead of slowing down, those nerves hit the gas. Sensing something is up that you need energy for, your pituitary gland gives you a shot of adrenaline. That's fine early in the day. But the half-life of caffeine is about six hours. So if you drink a 200-milligram mug of java at 3 p.m., you still have a shot's worth of espresso kicking around at 9 p.m. That's not conducive to sleep. Try to avoid caffeine after 2 p.m.—or at least make it a small cup.

MANAGING STRESS FOR GOOD SLEEP

Have you caught on yet that managing stress is a key component to feeling and performing your best through menopause? It's also essential for sleep. Again, because your hormones aren't helping (quite the opposite), you need to step in and give your body some extra assistance.

TAKE A DEEP BREATH: Honestly, one of the most easily accessible techniques to lower your stress throughout the day is deep breathing exercises. The North American Menopause Society recommends practicing this simple method throughout the day:

Sit in a straight-backed chair with both feet on the floor.

Rest your hands on your abdomen.

Slowly count to four while inhaling through your nose and feeling your abdomen rise.

Hold that breath for a second.

Then slowly count to four while exhaling through your mouth and letting your abdomen slowly fall.

Repeat this exercise five to ten times.

This type of deep breathing activates the vagus nerve and helps you move out of a sympathetic (fight-or-flight) state and triggers parasympathetic (rest-and-digest) activity. Practicing this type of breathing, pulling breath deep into your abdomen, while you're in child's pose can give you the double benefits of improving your pelvic floor health and reducing the risk or incidence of urinary incontinence while also reducing stress.

STRIKE A YOGA POSE: Yoga for relaxation is good for menopausal women. A 2013 study published in the *American Journal of Obstetrics and Gynecology* found that menopausal women who took a yoga class every week and practiced 20 minutes a day on their own had fewer hot flashes, better sex lives, and improved quality of life. Another study published in 2014 in *Menopause* failed to find benefits for hot flashes in a group of mostly postmenopausal women who did 12 weeks of yoga, but they slept better, with less insomnia, than those who didn't.

PRACTICE MINDFUL MEDITATION: Meditation has been used for centuries in religion as a form of prayer to connect with God and the universe. It is also widely used secularly to calm the mind and stay in the present, rather than allowing the brain to race with regret over the past or fret about the future. Practiced regularly, meditation is good for your mental and physical health, and it just may ease menopause symptoms and allow you to rest and recover better.

A study published in *Menopause* found that when a group of women experiencing at least seven moderate to severe hot flashes a day attended eight weekly mindfulness stress reduction classes, their hot flashes decreased by 40 percent. They also reported a significant increase in their quality of life.

Apps like Headspace offer structured meditation sessions to talk you through the process and help you with mindfulness, relaxation, and sleep.

SLEEP SUPPORT SUPPLEMENTS

The goal of this book is to help you work with your changing physiology by showing you where you can fill the gaps that your dwindling hormones are leaving behind. Sometimes you can do that by changing your training, diet, and lifestyle, and sometimes you need extra assistance.

I'm not a fan of sleeping pills, as they can be habit-forming and sometimes have side effects like daytime grogginess and sleepwalking. (And buying stuff in your sleep! A friend of Selene's once ordered a number of bike saddles in the middle of the night after taking Ambien and had no idea until they all started arriving.) I prefer more natural approaches. First, I encourage you to go back to the adaptogens discussed in chapter 4, as many of those products, such as ashwagandha and Holy Basil, are effective for reducing stress and promoting sleep. If adaptogens are not getting the job done, you can also try:

MELATONIN: A hormone produced in the pineal gland of the brain, melatonin is critical for your natural sleep-wake cycle. It seems logical that if you can't get to sleep, taking melatonin should help. If temperature-related sleep issues continue after you start taking it, try the smallest effective dose of melatonin, 0.3 to 1.0 milligrams, 30 minutes before bed.

Melatonin's role in sleep is a bit complex, however, and just taking a melatonin pill doesn't work the same way as melatonin that is naturally produced along with your other hormones. It can also have a "hangover" effect, keeping you groggy long after you've woken up for the day. I would recommend using valerian and tart cherry juice first, as these have been shown to naturally increase the body's production of melatonin and do not have the melatonin hangover side effect that is common when taking straight melatonin.

MONTMORENCY TART CHERRY JUICE CONCENTRATE: Tart cherry juice is high in the sleep-promoting chemical melatonin, enhances your body's own production of melatonin, and has anti-inflammatory properties (inflammation can disrupt sleep). It's also rich in antioxidants and polyphenols, so it checks all the boxes for what you need for the reparation process as you sleep. It also has a good track record. Research shows that older women (and men) slept better and for longer when they drank tart cherry juice before bed. For the best results, drink an ice-cold glass 30 minutes before bed to help your core temperature drop and send you into slumber.

VALERIAN ROOT (TEA OR CAPSULES): Some studies find that 400 to 600 milligrams of valerian extract before bed can improve sleep, including better sleep quality and making it easier to fall asleep faster.

Valerian can be a good complement to melatonin if you're using that supplement. Melatonin enhances deep sleep, whereas valerian can help you fall asleep faster.

BLACK COHOSH: Black cohosh (formally known as both *Actaea racemosa* and *Cimicifuga racemosa*), a member of the buttercup family, is a perennial plant that is native to North America. It has been widely studied as an alternative to menopausal hormone therapy for the alleviation of hot flashes and other menopausal symptoms. It can be taken as a supplement or a tea. Using black cohosh can be beneficial in improving sleep quality by reducing hot flashes, but it should only be used for four to six months and definitely not more than six, because of its slight potential to cause liver damage. The calming adaptogens listed earlier are a better choice.

SMART RECOVERY PRACTICES

Sleep is a big part of the recovery picture, but there are many ways in which you can accelerate the process. These "active recovery" techniques are updated from *ROAR* for the menopausal athlete and are useful immediately after hard workouts and in the days following challenging sessions when you wake up feeling like someone poured sludge into your muscles. You may not feel like moving, but getting the blood circulating through active recovery will make you feel better.

COOLING DOWN: Many athletes I work with are diligent about warming up before a workout or race but often blow off the cool-down because they're in a hurry or they don't see the value. If you're one of these people, take just two or three minutes—it doesn't take long—to properly cool down. This is the first part of your recovery process.

By continuing to move at an easy, relaxed pace, you allow your body to quickly drop your heart rate and start to shift your blood distribution. If you go from full sprint to full stop, the blood pools in your legs, which can not only make you feel dizzy but also stall the recovery process, because it limits your ability to get key nutrients into your muscle cells so they can repair. Maintaining the blood flow back and forth from your muscles with a proper cool-down enhances nutrient exchange and muscle repair. This is especially advantageous when you have two workouts in one day, as many triathletes do, or when you have an evening session followed by an early-morning workout the next day. Cooling down is especially important for women, because we experience a greater decrease in arterial blood pressure after exercise than men.

COLD BATHS: After exercise, there are normal changes in blood pressure and blood-flow fluctuations, and it takes longer than usual for core body temperature to return to normal—especially in women, who have a harder time off-loading heat post-exercise. In peri- and postmenopausal women, blood vessel compliance is also an issue; their blood vessels are less responsive to changes in constriction and dilation, increasing the time it takes for the hot blood of the muscles to be pulled away and drop their core temperature. Women have a natural post-exercise response to vasodilate and divert more blood to their skin—and away from their muscles—to try to cool themselves; this is exacerbated in the postmenopause state, which can cause unwanted post-exercise "head rushes" (blood pressure dropping too far). With less blood circulating to and from your muscles, you remain in a prolonged stressed state with more metabolic waste lingering in your muscles, increasing inflammation.

Cooling your body in a cold tub can trick your body into redistributing the blood from the skin back into circulation through the muscles. You may have heard that diving into a cool pool or taking an ice bath can stall your recovery and increase muscle soreness. This may indeed be a fact for men, because their blood vessels naturally constrict post-exercise to push blood away from the skin and back into central circulation. When men take a post-exercise plunge into cold water, they can start shivering and get microspasms in their already fatigued muscles, which can lead to soreness and stalled recovery. This is not the case for women, who need assistance speeding up vasoconstriction after hard exertion. So ladies, the ice bath is here to stay!

ACTIVE RECOVERY EXERCISE: On rest days, it's a good idea to do some *very* easy exercise rather than sink into a chair for the day. This is especially important for menopausal women, who tell me that they now actually do much worse with complete days off and need to keep moving to stay limber and feel fresh. Active recovery does not have to be sport-specific. It can be any activity you like, so long as it is really, truly *very easy.* Many women set out with the intention of doing active recovery and end up pushing a little on the hills or picking up the pace. This prevents their muscles from fully recovering.

On your rest days, you want to increase your circulation, which will help your muscles repair without challenging them and prolonging the damage. Take a walk, go for an easy ride to get coffee, do some easy laps in the pool, or perform some yin yoga. Keep it short and sweet—about 45 minutes to an hour is all you need.

MASSAGE: Professional athletes have massage therapists for a reason—it speeds up the recovery process. Massage flushes your muscles, so you push out the fluid that carries the waste products of muscle breakdown and make way for fresh, nutrient-rich blood to come in and help repair and rebuild. Massage also breaks up the adhesions (knots) that can form from overuse, so your muscles work more smoothly and painlessly. Research shows that massage can help prevent delayed onset muscle soreness (DOMS).

In one study, researchers had volunteers push out reps on the leg press machine until their quads and hamstrings flew the white surrender flag. Then half of the participants got a massage while the other half hobbled home. The lucky participants who received the massage rated their post-exercise soreness to be a five on a one to ten scale, while the exercise-only group rated their pain at nearly a nine. And these weren't just subjective impressions—the massage group also enjoyed better blood flow (a sign of recovery, since exercise-induced muscle injury reduces blood flow). In fact, the massage group had improved blood flow for up to 72 hours after their rubdown. The exercise-only group had compromised circulation for more than 48 hours, returning to normal after 72 hours.

Even if you're not a pro and can't afford a massage every time you need or want one, there's no need to suffer for days. With the right tools and techniques, you can do a pretty good job yourself. Massage guns like Theragun and Hypervolt work like a charm. You can also do easy, inexpensive self-massage with rubber balls and foam balls. See "Work Out the Knots" in the following chapter for self-massage techniques you can perform with a few simple recovery tools. For the best results, do these moves as soon as you can after a hard workout.

COMPRESSION PUMPS: If you follow any pro athletes on Instagram, you're bound to see some shots of them, legs up, encased in what look like giant, inflated boots. That's pretty much exactly what they are. Compression pumps are simply zip-on leg sleeves (often, but not always, with feet attached) that attach to a motorized pump. They inflate and deflate in a systematic way to compress and flush your muscles. So a deep squeeze from your feet to your groin pushes fluids out and reduces blood flow in. Then the blood flows back into the muscles when the sleeves release to significantly increase tissue oxygenation, nutrient exchange, and metabolic waste removal.

NormaTec was the original name in compression pumps, or recovery pumps, but now there are a number of players, including RecoveryPump, Game Ready, and Elevated Legs. Some of these products combine pneumatic compression with circulating cool water. The cooling-compression combination is particularly good for women, as it can help counteract the vasodilation response that women experience and enhance blood flow to the muscles. Cooling-compression is also ideal for joint inflammation or soft-tissue injury that involves swelling. Because women's blood flow naturally takes longer to normalize post-exercise, they should use compression pumps within 30 minutes of finishing a workout or race, whereas men can wait a bit longer (60 to 90 minutes) to garner the benefits.

ELECTRICAL MUSCLE STIMULATION DEVICES: Electrical muscle stimulation (EMS) devices allow you to get the benefits of active recovery without moving a muscle—sort of. When you attach the electrodes to your muscles and turn the machine on, the electronic muscle stimulation triggers rhythmic muscle contractions (which is pretty freaky at first) while you're not doing a thing. There are various EMS devices on the market, including Marc Pro, PowerDot, and Compex. The Compex and PowerDot use a traditional EMS program that delivers a strong, static contraction with a sudden release. The Marc Pro employs a moderate contraction with a slow release. Both types are great at simulating active recovery and enhancing blood flow to tight, bound areas of muscle, but some experts believe that the Marc Pro may be more suitable for muscle recovery (or for those with chronic pain) because it allows fluids to flow in and out of the muscle cells without the undue fatigue that some people experience with traditional EMS systems.

Pneumatic compression and muscle stimulation products carry a fairly high price tag. But if you're an athlete who already invests in a coach and regular massages, it could be worth a look.

COMPRESSION GARMENTS: Whether you're an endurance or power athlete, chances are you already have a pair of compression socks or tights. Nurses and other workers who spend long hours on their feet have been wearing these for decades to assist blood flow from the lower extremities back to the heart. Worn after exercise, they may improve blood oxygen levels and subsequent recovery. The science isn't definitive on how well these garments work, but research suggests that they can lessen swelling, fatigue, and muscle soreness after intense exercise. One study published in the *Journal of Strength and Conditioning Research* reported that women and men who wore compression socks for 48 hours after running a marathon improved their performance on a treadmill test two weeks later.

NEXT LEVEL MENOPAUSE MAKEOVER:
KEEPING A 60+ TRIATHLETE IN THE GAME

LISA,* 62, is a vegan 70.3 Ironman distance athlete who is struggling with muscle loss and poor recovery. She wants to turn that around so she can be competitive in her age group again.

GENERAL ASSESSMENT

Lisa is in generally good shape. She's 5'4", 134 pounds and 24 percent body fat. She's not really looking to lose weight, but she would like to get stronger by building and maintaining muscle mass. She's also really struggling with poor recovery. She feels like her training and performance is flat; she fades in the run and her lower back starts to hurt, and she's stuck in this gray zone where she's not making any progress.

She has been a vegan athlete for about 15 years. She feels like she's getting enough protein, but when I probe a little further, I learn that she's relying pretty heavily on ultra-processed meat alternatives like Tofurky and other "faux meats" that are really not providing as much protein as she thinks, and also are low in important amino acids like leucine.

On her longer running and cycling days, she has been suffering with some bloating and GI issues and is having trouble eating, even after she's done. Those processed foods are not very good for the gut, so some of her GI issues may be coming from those. She also doesn't have a strong sense of thirst, so she says she ends up getting progressively dehydrated at times.

As with many triathletes, she does a lot of double workout training days. She's doing a lot of moderate to hard intensity work and not much, if any, recovery days. The group rides are unpredictable hammerfests. The swimming sessions are not easy. The run is her weaker sport, so that's always a little hard, even on the easier days. We need to adjust her schedule to gain some balance; improve lean mass development, and get her out of this constant stressful, catabolic state. We need to make a few tweaks to be sure she's getting the quality training she needs.

That means adding a lifting program. She needs to be strong to be able to complete the 70.3 distance well, and to feel good as she's going through the training. Doing just sort-of-hard sessions are making her weaker and more tired.

We also need to adjust her diet and improve the quantity and quality of her protein intake so when she is performing anabolic strength exercise, she can generate that lean muscle mass. Right now she uses pea-based protein powder, but that does not contain enough leucine to help with muscle protein synthesis for active women, so we boost the amino acid profile by adding fermented BCAAs, which guarantees they are vegan. We also include more real foods like beans and rice and pulse pastas to include more protein everywhere we can. Because I really want her to have a diverse, nutrient-dense diet, we add some "superfoods" including blue spirulina, chia and hemp seeds, ginger, and others. We make sure she develops good fueling habits by eating before and after training, so she has the carbs and protein she needs for energy and muscle synthesis.

HER NEW ROUTINE

Here's how her new schedule looks after our makeover:

MONDAY: This is a hard day. We keep the swim squad at 9 a.m. Then in the evening, she does some heavy lifting. Because she's new to lifting we phase it in by starting with bodyweight and technique exercises. Then we start adding weights and getting progressively heavier as she gains strength and confidence.

TUESDAY: Another hard day. We keep the hill work on the bike, but she goes with a faster friend who she chases up the hill or has them chase her to get in that real race simulation intensity that is specific to her cycling needs.

WEDNESDAY: Easy day. We keep swim squad, but no track session. She can go for a super easy run just to shake out her legs if she wants.

THURSDAY: Moderate to hard. She does a warm-up ride to the gym, then she potentiates her posterior chain (think glutes, hamstrings, postural muscles) and core with a heavy lifting session in the gym, then she goes out for hard hill work on the bike right after, drilling in that specificity.

FRIDAY: Hard day. Open water swimming in the morning. In the afternoon, she does an easy 30 minute run then finishes that run with 4 rounds of kettlebell swings and lunges and box jumps with equipment at home.

SATURDAY: Super easy day. We skip the club session and just opt for a 2 to 3 hour super easy, Zone 1 endurance ride that she can do with friends if she wants, but it needs to be cruisy and fun. To really enforce the Zone 1, we keep her at a specific RPE of 3 to 4, where she is almost soft pedaling any small rise in the road.

SUNDAY: Easy play day. Open water swimming if she wants. But otherwise just a chill day to let all the super hard resistance training work sink in so she can really build that strength before she increases volume as she gets closer to her race.

COMING BACK FROM INJURY

You've been in this game long enough to know that whether you race cyclocross, trail-run, line up at tris, snowboard down mountainsides, or push yourself in the CrossFit box, torn muscles, sprained ankles, broken bones, and the like are an inevitable part of the game. As we get older, recovery can take longer, but you can take measures to help your body heal more quickly so you can get back to what you love sooner.

As a menopausal woman, you want to limit muscle loss as much as possible, but that can be a challenge when you're laid up and unable to exercise the way you usually do. Injuries and surgery create hormonal and inflammatory stress that trigger rapid muscle loss. You can lose nearly a pound of muscle mass during the first two weeks of being laid up with a single immobilized limb, and that loss is worsened by metabolic changes that reduce your ability to build muscle. You also experience strength loss related not to muscle loss but to disuse. Finally, you lose the skeletal calcium and magnesium stores that are necessary for muscle contractions. In general, you lose strength three times as fast as you lose muscle following an injury that leaves you immobilized. Again, you're already losing muscle contraction strength during this time of life, so minimizing this loss is important.

The first step is adjusting your diet to slow the rate of muscle loss by getting enough protein. Make sure to eat 0.9 to 1.1 grams per pound of body weight, or 126 to 154 grams for a 140-pound woman. This diet won't eliminate muscle loss completely, but it will slow it down. For the best results, choose a protein that is easily absorbed and contains the right amino acids to stimulate muscle growth. For example, whey protein, which is more rapidly digested and absorbed than soy or casein, has been shown to be more anabolic. It is also richer in the BCAA leucine, which stimulates muscle protein synthesis; you need even more of this amino acid if you've been injured.

High-stress exercise, post-exercise muscle damage, and injuries all change amino acid and protein metabolism in your muscles and increase the metabolism of leucine. The damage in the muscle tissue stimulates the breakdown of BCAAs (and total muscle-cell breakdown). To stop that breakdown and promote recovery, you need to increase the levels of leucine in those tissues. The more leucine you take in, the more quickly your body begins to send out signals to make muscle. For the best results, aim to take in 30 grams of protein that contain about 3 grams of leucine three times a day. Good injury-recovery foods include lean meat, low-fat Greek yogurt, and nut butter on sprouted grain bread.

Keep in mind that this isn't the time to pull out the traditional recovery drinks formulated with carbohydrates, which stimulate insulin release and generally work with leucine to improve muscle building. When you're in a state of anabolic resistance, such as after an injury, adding carbs slows the rate at which the protein is digested and absorbed and does not improve the rate of muscle synthesis. What you need now is primarily protein.

You can make your muscles more reactive to the muscle-building effects of the amino acids found in protein by also including omega-3 fatty acids, like the kind found in fish oil. Take about 4 grams a day while you're recovering.

To put it all together, imagine a hypothetical 140-pound woman who wipes out on her bike and ends up with a broken collarbone and significant muscle bruising. To reduce muscle-mass loss and preserve strength during her recovery, the ideal recommended daily protein intake is 126 to 154 grams of protein, ideally spread across four main meals (40 grams per meal with 2 to 3 grams of leucine and 15 to 20 grams with snacks) eaten every three to five hours. This amount counteracts the anabolic resistance caused by her injuries, and the equal timing keeps her muscle synthesis rates elevated over a 24-hour period. A split supplementation of 4 grams of omega-3 fatty acids (2 grams in the morning, 2 grams before bed) will maintain the upturn of muscle synthesis signaling.

Accidents and crashes happen. But knowing how to manipulate your body's responses to minimize muscle and strength loss will shorten the recovery time and get you back in the game sooner.

14

STABILITY, MOBILITY, AND CORE STRENGTH: KEEP YOUR FOUNDATION STRONG

Move pain-free through menopause and beyond.

Lifting heavy sh*t can stem the muscle and strength loss that comes as our estrogen levels decline, taking our lean muscle mass with it. But you can't lift heavy sh*t without good stability, mobility, and a strong core—all of which are also impacted as hormones fluctuate and eventually flatline.

Women generate most of their strength and stability through their hips. Though we tend to have powerful lower-body muscles, our core muscles are relatively weak by comparison. That's why, when you watch some women perform a squat or jump down from a box, you see their knees caving in. The core stabilizing muscles in their hips and glutes are asleep at the wheel.

This weakness sets us up for ligament tears and other orthopedic injuries, even in our premenopausal years. In our menopausal years, it also can contribute to trouble with urinary incontinence, because there's too much pressure and uneven force being applied to our pelvic floor muscles, making it difficult for them to function properly and prevent urine from leaking out.

As mentioned in chapter 3, estrogen can loosen your connective tissues, while progesterone increases the tension in your tendons and ligaments. As those hormones swing during perimenopause and eventually completely drop off postmenopause, we can find ourselves literally destabilized, having lost connective tissue integrity as well as muscle mass.

Many women also suffer from what is sometimes erroneously called "menopause arthritis" as inflammation rises and causes them to feel more aches, pains, and unhealthy stiffness through their joints. They may also feel more muscle tension than they used to. That's because higher levels of cortisol can make their muscles feel tight and fatigued.

If you struggle with debilitating joint pain that makes it difficult, if not impossible, to exercise, talk to your doctor about menopausal hormone therapy. Research has connected low levels of estradiol (E2), progesterone, and testosterone with increased knee swelling and other osteoarthritis-related structural changes in women. (Researchers say that this points to an explanation for the sex differences in osteoarthritis: men do not experience these structural changes.) Research on more than 10,000 postmenopausal women, as part of the Women's Health Initiative, also reported that women on estrogen therapy experienced a modest but sustained reduction in joint pain.

All menopausal women should practice some mobility and stability exercises as part of their daily routine. This chapter will show you what you need to know.

STABILITY AND MOBILITY FROM THE GROUND UP

Stability and mobility are two sides of the same coin. When you have good stability, you can move quickly and powerfully, with greater ease and with less risk of injury. Having good mobility—being able to move your body the way you want without being restricted by too much stiffness or by imbalances—makes you more stable, because you can adjust as needed and catch yourself when you're knocked off balance.

You want just enough tension in your joints to provide support and stability as you're lifting heavy sh*t, without too much stiffness that will impair your range of motion and make you more prone to developing injury and imbalance.

Women's joints in particular are prone to being too lax. This happens because they've been stretched out over time, says Kelly Starrett, my good friend, one of the premier mobility experts in the world, and author of *Becoming a Supple Leopard*.

As he explained in *ROAR*, "When your tissues are more lax, your joints don't have the integrity they should because they're stretched out. This also impairs your proprioception, the sense of where your limbs are in space and in relation to one another, which is a huge factor in mobility and stability." (It's also incredibly important to preventing falls when we reach older age.) When you're not getting proper proprioceptive feedback, your movement patterns are thrown off, which is a problem when you're trying to lift heavy sh*t and do plyometrics.

"A stiff athlete leans into the stiffness for support as they move," he continues. "When you're hypermobile, you have to actually know the end of your range of motion in a conscious way."

Your spine plays an essential role in your stability as well. And being a woman, you face some inherent challenges with spinal stability. For one, as explained in *ROAR*, everyone's lumbar spine has some wedge-shaped vertebrae—similar to the wedge-shaped bricks or stones that architects use to create arches—that form the natural curvature of the spine. Well, we women are blessed with one additional wedge—three instead of the two that our male counterparts get—so that, should we get pregnant, we can lean back further (up to 28 degrees) for stability and keep our center of gravity in our hips as our pregnant belly grows larger.

In some women, this swayback posture becomes permanent as the spine-supporting muscles get stretched. This exaggerated lumbar curvature tips your pelvis forward and starts inhibiting muscles in your trunk and pelvic floor, which can trigger incontinence problems, especially in menopause, when your pelvic floor begins to weaken from loss of estrogen.

At this point, you also may be experiencing some lifelong stability alterations from habitually wearing high heels if you've been in a professional setting that required that style of dress. As Starrett explains, high heels tip your body forward, forcing you to adapt your posture by leaning back (and taking advantage of that third wedge). Spend enough hours (or at this point, years) in wedges and pumps, and your body adapts to that posture permanently. And it's not just your spine. Having your heels lifted so much of the time also impacts your ankles.

"Women who wear high heels most of the time end up with shorter heel cords, which in turn prevents the ankle from rotating and moving through its full range of motion when you're not in high heels," Starrett explains. "You start to walk and strike the ground with your feet turned out to accommodate the shortened heel cord." One 2010 study reported that women who wore heels two inches or higher five or more days a week had calf muscles that were an average of 13 percent shorter and Achilles' tendons that were significantly thicker than those of their peers who opted for flats most of the time.

Because your feet are fixed in a downward position, you don't have the same heel-to-toe rolling motion you do with regular shoes, so you aren't able to push off the ground very well. Your hip flexors step in to help move you forward, but that can cause them to become short and tight, further exacerbating the increased curvature in your lower back. Following the mobility plan in this chapter will help undo some of the damage, but you also need to ditch the heels.

Finally, as an active woman of menopausal age, you've probably been in the game for quite a few years, if not decades. That means a lot of repetitive movements . . . and the inflammation, tensions, and adhesions that can come with them. Knotted muscles decrease your mobility (and therefore your stability) and cause discomfort. Breaking up the adhesions and scar tissue within your muscles and the fascia that cover your muscles can improve your comfort and mobility.

WORK OUT THE KNOTS

Starrett shares some of his key moves for breaking up adhesions and improving mobility in *ROAR*. He expands on that here in *NEXT LEVEL* because, as he says, "at this point, women need more soft tissue work to maintain total and complete range of motion."

I couldn't agree more. With the loss of collagen and lean muscle mass during the menopausal years, along with more systemic inflammation, maintaining mobility is critical. Otherwise, you develop tension and adhesions or muscle knots that decrease your mobility and cause discomfort. Erin Carson seconds that "motion," so to speak. "You can't skip the tissue care and mobility work at this point. It's what sets the stage for the strength and power and higher-intensity work you need," she says. And she should know. As mentioned previously, Erin set an Ironman 70.3 personal best time (by nearly 20 minutes!) at age 53 by taking her own advice.

You don't need fancy equipment. A foam roller or a pair of lacrosse or tennis balls stuffed in a sock are excellent tools and can help compress and massage stuck spots. Breaking up the adhesions and scar tissue within the muscle and the fascia that covers the muscle allows for greater mobility. If you lie on a lacrosse ball or foam roller and it hurts, those are tissues that aren't gliding correctly, says Starrett. "Normal healthy muscles shouldn't hurt during compression."

By rolling your muscles, you can smooth out those spots with compression. But note—and this is important—if you press so hard that you have to hold your breath, you're going too deep and triggering your fight-or-flight response, which will only exacerbate the problem. Press into the roller or ball with just enough pressure that it's slightly uncomfortable, but not painful. This will send a signal to the central nervous system to reduce tension, which relieves soreness and improves range of motion.

Here are a few excellent foam roller and lacrosse ball moves that hit the hips, lower back, Achilles' tendon, and foot regions, all of which tend to get tight and knotted. These moves are especially good for menopausal women. Roll until you feel relief in your tight or tender spots in about a minute or so.

PLANTAR ROLL

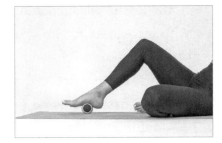

Place your foot on top of a lacrosse ball and press down to apply pressure as you roll along the length of your foot and back to relieve tightness in the plantar fascia. For better precision, you can use a golf ball.

CALF SMASH

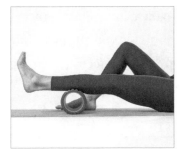

Place your left calf on top of your roller. Relax your muscles and sink into the roller. Then slowly roll your lower leg from side to side, kneading your way into the tissues. Contract and relax the calf by flexing and extending your foot through its full range of motion. Switch legs.

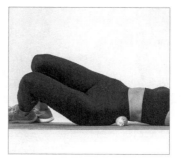

Place two lacrosse balls in a sock and twist the sock between the balls to create space between them. Lie on the floor with your knees bent, feet flat on the floor. Lift your hips and place the balls beneath your lower back at the base of your lumbar spine, so that each ball is on either side of your spine. Lower your back down, but keep your hips off the floor. Drop your left knee toward your right side and rotate your hips slightly to the right, making sure that your shoulders stay in contact with the floor. Then rotate your hips to the opposite side. Rotate from side to side until you feel the tension release. Then move up to the next vertebra and repeat, continuing this sequence to the top of the lumbar spine (where your lower-back curve ends).

GLUTE SMASH

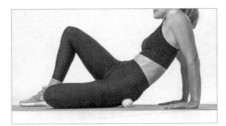

Sit on the floor with your knees bent and position a lacrosse ball on the side of your left hip. Press into the ball with your hip (slightly under your butt) and drop your left knee out toward the floor. Slowly roll from side to side across your glute. If you come across a particularly painful area, contract and relax and keep applying gentle pressure to release the tissue. Return to center and repeat on the opposite side.

ADDUCTOR SMASH

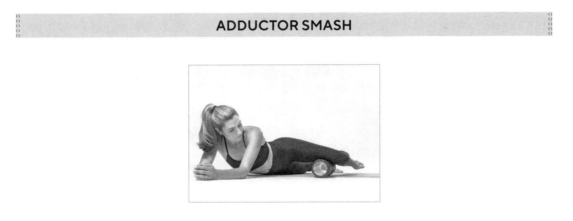

Lie facedown on a cushioned surface, bend your left leg to the side and place your roller on the inside of your thigh. Relax your muscles to sink into the roller. Drive your right hip toward the floor to deepen the pressure. Move the roller along the muscle to check for tight spots. Repeat the process on your left side.

QUAD ROLL

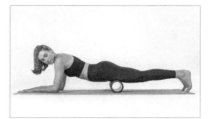

Lie facedown on the floor and place a foam roller under your hips. Lean on your left leg and roll up and down the front of your thigh from your hip to your knee. Switch legs.

ANTERIOR HIP SMASH

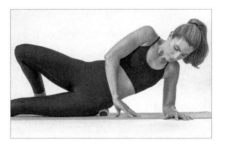

Place the ball at the top of your left hip bone. Press your body weight into the ball and then roll back and forth. Then relax and rotate your femur to add twisting forces into the move.

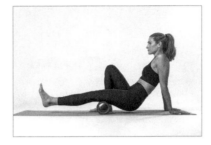

Sit with your left hamstring on the roller; bend your right knee and place your right foot on the floor. Place your hands on the floor behind you and roll up and down from your knee to just under your left butt cheek. Switch legs and repeat.

OPEN UP THE RESTRICTED SPOTS

These moves from Erin Carson are designed to open up the areas that are especially tight in women, such as the hips, shoulders, and chest. They also glide your joints through a range of multidirectional motion to get (and keep) your body ready for activity. For the best results, do these moves after you exercise to work out the knots with your foam rolling and soft tissue work. Or start with a few foam-rolling moves, particularly calves, outer glutes, and hips.

SI JOINT GLIDE

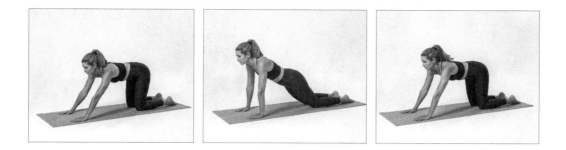

On a cushioned surface, assume a tabletop position on your hands and knees. Press your hips back toward your heels, until your legs are bent about 45 degrees. Then press your hips forward and down until your body is almost diagonal to the floor. Repeat, gliding back and forth 16 times.

FOAM ROLL WITH LAT ROTATION

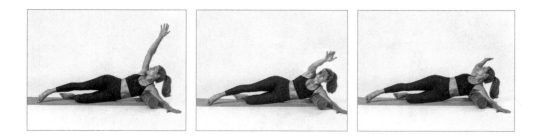

Lie on your left side, left leg in front of the right for support, with a foam roller under your arm, supporting your lats, and your left arm extended, resting on the floor. Reach toward the ceiling with your right arm. Then rotate your torso forward and lower your outstretched arm toward the floor. Rotate back, reaching the arm slightly behind you. Continue rotating for 10 repetitions to the front and 10 to the back.

LAT GLIDING

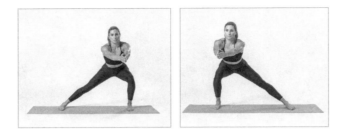

Stand with your legs in a straddle stance, arms outstretched in front of you, palms together. Squat back so your legs are bent 45 degrees. Keeping your upper body stable, straighten your right leg and lunge to the left side. Then reverse the move and straighten your left leg and lunge to the right side. Repeat back and forth 10 times to each side.

LATERAL STEP AND REACH

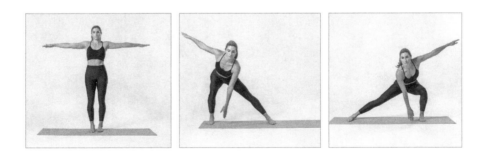

Stand with your feet together, arms outstretched to the sides. Lunge to the right with your right foot, bending the right knee while simultaneously reaching across your body and touching the inside of the right foot with your left hand. Return to start. Repeat for five reps and then switch sides.

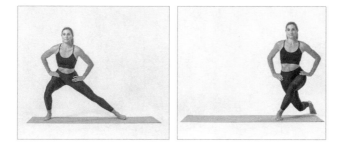

Stand with your feet together, arms at your side, elbows slightly bent. Step to the right and dip into a 45-degree lunge. Then push off and step back, bringing your right leg behind your left, and dip into a 45-degree diagonal lunge. Repeat stepping to the side and diagonally back for five repetitions. Then switch sides.

KICK UP YOUR CORE WORK

Your core is more than your abs; it's everything but your limbs. Strengthening your core not only protects your joints, which are more vulnerable as estrogen and progesterone decline, but also prevents or mitigates urinary incontinence. Put the following basic moves in your menopausal core arsenal.

WINDSHIELD WIPERS

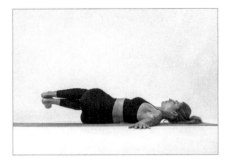

Lie on your back with your knees bent and your feet off the floor so that your thighs are perpendicular and your calves are parallel to the floor. Extend your arms out to the sides, palms facing down. Keeping your shoulders on the floor, slowly drop your legs to the left until they touch the floor. Return to start. Repeat on the opposite side.

PLANK

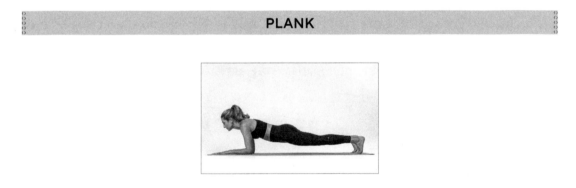

Lie facedown on the floor with your upper body propped on your forearms with your elbows directly beneath your shoulders. Your torso should be up off the floor so your body is in a straight line, supported by your forearms and toes. Your back should not arch or droop. Hold 10 to 20 seconds.

SHOULDER BRIDGE

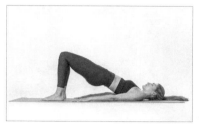

Lie on your back with your knees bent and feet flat on the floor, hip-width apart. Keeping your thighs parallel, contract your glutes and lift your hips toward the ceiling so that your body forms a straight line from your shoulders to your knees. Rest your arms at your sides, palms down, or intensify the move by clasping your hands beneath you. Hold for a few seconds. Lower and repeat.

SUPERMAN

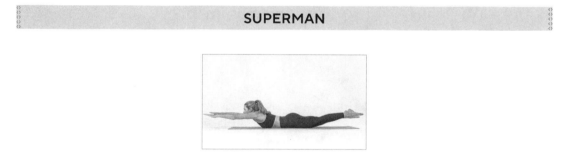

Lie face down on the floor, arms fully extended in front of you, palms down. Squeeze your glutes and simultaneously raise your arms, legs, and chest off the floor and hold for two seconds. Lower your arms, legs, and chest back to the starting position and repeat. *Note*: You can make this move easier to start by lifting just one arm and leg at a time, alternating sides throughout the set.

SWEEPING SIDE PLANK

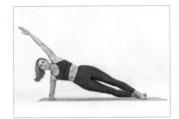

Sit on your right hip with legs extended to the side, knees slightly bent. Cross your left foot in front of the right. Place your right hand on the floor directly beneath your shoulder. Place your left hand on your left leg. Lift your hips off the floor, extending your left arm overhead so that your body forms a diagonal line. Without bending your right arm, lower your hips and left arm back to start. Repeat for 30 seconds. Switch sides.

V-UP

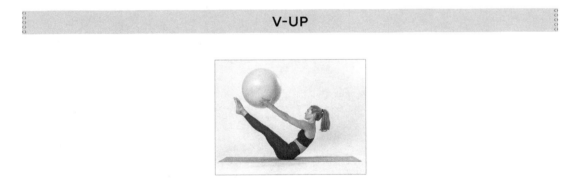

Holding a stability ball between your hands, lie on your back with your arms extended straight up toward the ceiling, so that the ball is above your chest; your legs are extended and your feet pointed. Contract your abs and simultaneously lift your torso and legs, so that your body forms a V and the ball and your feet meet above your hips. Pause, then return to the starting position.

15

MOTIVATION AND THE MENTAL GAME: YOUR MIND MATTERS

Keep your mojo running during menopause.

I thought I was finished."

Those were the words of Lynda Rowan, a dual citizen of both Australia and the United States who has competed in Sprint, Olympic, 70.3, and Ironman triathlons and has represented both countries at the ITU (International Triathlon Union) World Age Group Championships. She's also been an endurance coach for 30 years. Out of the blue, after one of her long runs, she was walking back to her car and thought, *I don't want to do this anymore.*

Lynda had lost her mojo for the sport she'd loved for more than three decades seemingly overnight. She wasn't alone. We hear this all the time. Women describe that moment as a spark just going out. Their heart isn't in it. They've gone from waking up to hit the pool for a Masters swim at 5:30 a.m. to having no motivation to work out at all, let alone before sunrise.

Lynda took a break and eventually found her way back, now realizing that what she was experiencing were menopausal doldrums—her motivation going MIA when her sex hormones began messing with her brain. Not all women come back from the doldrums. That's one reason we're writing this book—to help women stay in sport when mood swings, body composition changes, body image issues, and other menopause transition symptoms make them just want to throw in the towel.

THIS IS YOUR BRAIN ON MENOPAUSE

It's pretty clear that menopause can wreak havoc on your mental health and make you feel off your game. For one, your brain chemistry is changing. During the transition to menopause, decreasing estrogen levels alter your memory circuitry function and performance, according to a study published in the *Journal of Neuroscience.*

Estrogen also helps with the maintenance and regulation of network integrity within your brain, sort of like the bucket truck crews that roam the neighborhood making sure that your cable lines are all connected. When estrogen declines, you lose some bucket trucks, especially in the hippocampus and its related structures—areas of the brain that play a major role in memory, learning, and emotion regulation. As a result, memory, cognition, and attention suffer.

The loss of brain-derived neurotrophic factor is partially to blame. BDNF is closely associated with brain function. One study of more than 200 women ages 45 to 55 reported that BDNF levels were associated with verbal and associative memory (the ability to remember the name of someone you just met) in postmenopausal women. When levels are low, brain fog follows. That's because estrogen interacts with BDNF in the brain to promote neuron health. Both estrogen and BDNF stimulate neurogenesis (the creation of new neurons) in the hippocampus. As estrogen fluctuates and declines, your brain loses that stimulus. BDNF also naturally declines with age, so that can be a double whammy for menopausal women.

As mentioned earlier, estrogen fluctuations and decline can lead to mood swings and feelings of panic, anxiety, or anger. Not to mention the frustration and low mood that can accompany bouts of brain fog.

Topping off these mental challenges is an icing of negative body image issues.

The physical (and mental) changes that can accompany menopause and that come with age, such as changing body composition, thinning skin and hair, vaginal dryness, and issues with sex drive, can take a toll on your self-esteem, confidence, and body image.

A survey of more than 1,800 women over age 50 published in the *Journal of Women & Aging* highlighted the emotional minefield that many women find themselves navigating during their menopausal years. As one woman put it:

> *I am ashamed of my aging body and ashamed that I am ashamed. I believe women pay an enormous price for cultural biases related to gender and age—58 years*

This 58-year-old woman is not alone. Another recent study indicated that just 12 percent of older women are satisfied with their body size. Roughly 80 percent of women in the United States reported being dissatisfied with how their bodies look, according to an online survey conducted by Ipsos on behalf of RiverMend Health. It's common for even normal and healthy weight women to want to be thinner and to diet. Feelings like these can set up a vicious, worsening cycle of depression and anxiety, as negative body image has been linked to both in menopausal women.

All of this can wreak havoc on your mojo, motivation, and mental game during your menopausal years. But don't shut this book in despair. Just as you can work with your changing physiology to optimize your physical health, you also can train your brain to boost your confidence, improve your body image, lift your moods, and sharpen your mental game.

GET YOUR GROOVE BACK

Obviously, we are not professional psychotherapists, so before we start, we would urge any reader who is struggling with depression, crippling anxiety, and/or an eating disorder to please make a call to schedule an appointment with a professional who can provide the help you need.

Even though we're not psychotherapists, Selene and I do have decades of coaching experience, and my life's work has been devoted to helping women adapt to changing female physiology for optimum performance. So if you're just stuck in a menopause malaise like millions of other women, these strategies can help you get your groove back.

GO HARD: We outlined the importance of sprint interval training (SIT) for physical performance in chapter 5, but it bears repeating here because SIT also has mental health benefits. There's evidence that your body pumps out more BDNF when you do sprint interval training, and research shows that it helps improve cognition and working memory. In other words, SIT blows out that brain fog. Those increases in BDNF also can alleviate anxiety and depression and definitely make you feel better.

CHANGE YOUR TRAINING: This is important. All too often, when women find that their training isn't working like it used to after hitting their menopausal years, they immediately double down and do more of the same type of training (and sometimes start dieting to boot). But your body is different now. That means you need to train differently, even if you're doing the same sports. Any lifelong endurance athlete will tell you that, as they got older—especially women in menopause—they needed more truly easy days, more strength and mobility work, and more short, high-intensity workouts (like SIT), along with less overall volume. Less is more. Quality is everything. Trust the process here. You'll feel and perform better.

RETHINK YOUR RELATIONSHIP WITH WEIGHT: There's nothing wrong with wanting to improve your body composition by building strong muscles and losing some unwanted fat, but women often give the number on the scale too much power and influence over their lives. Pouring too much of your mental energy into hitting a magic number on the scale or a certain size on the clothing rack is counterproductive.

Thinking negatively about your weight day in and day out can keep you from feeling and performing your best. Also, contrary to what we tell ourselves, lighter is not always better. One woman's scale may say 132, but if she is proportionately low in lean muscle, being "lighter" is not "better." Likewise, another woman's scale may read 25 pounds heavier, but she's out there crushing in her triathlons because she is literally being powered by strong muscle mass.

In *ROAR*, I revealed my own journey with weight and performance. Years ago, I was a competitive cyclist and triathlete, racing XTERRA off-road triathlons at 136 pounds and a full Ironman at 147 pounds. Today I do mostly CrossFit-style workouts, gravel riding, and ocean swimming for fun at 128 pounds. That's a span of 19 pounds. Over the course of her mountain bike racing career, Selene had some of her best performances at 138 and worst at 127, even as she kept battling that nagging inner voice always telling her that lighter was better.

Recently retired cycling phenom Katie Compton, the most successful cyclocross racer (male or female) in the United States and the winner of more than 20 World Cups, also shared her story in *ROAR*. Despite being one of the most dominant racers ever, Compton struggled with body image and weight her entire life. At her heaviest she was 172, and at her lightest in the low 130s. But when she was restricting food and trying to stay at that low end, her health and performance deteriorated. She decided to step off the scale and eat when she was hungry and focus on being a powerful cyclist. That strategy worked.

It can be difficult for women of the "thin is in" generation to let go of the idea that skinnier is always better. The Kate Moss culture drilled it into us that our thighs shouldn't touch and our muscles shouldn't be big. Times have changed. Strong trumps skinny. Embrace this mindset.

This is especially beneficial if you participate in a sport, like cycling or running, that is power-to-weight-based, meaning that it rewards athletes who can produce a lot of power for every pound of body mass. Too often athletes get so fixated on the weight part of the equation that they forget about improving their performance by working on the other half—getting stronger and producing more power.

Getting stronger also improves your confidence and body image. One study of more than 340 women, average age of 62, found that participating in a strength training program significantly improved their body image, personal satisfaction, and health-related quality of life.

GET STRONG: Again, if you want your body to be a different weight so you can run or ride or perform your sport better, flip the script and start focusing on getting stronger rather than putting all the emphasis on getting lighter. By getting stronger, you'll feel and perform better, and that's more likely to favorably change your body composition and improve your physical, mental, and emotional health.

WRITE A POSITIVE SELF-TALK SCRIPT: There's a reason why people call negative talk like name-calling and heckling "trash talk": it's meant to trash your opponent's confidence by making them feel like, well, trash. Yet how often do we trash-talk ourselves and expect a different, somehow more positive, outcome? Negative self-talk produces anxiety. You don't need more anxiety. On the flip side, research shows that positive, motivational self-talk improves performance and can even make exercise feel easier. Create a positive self-talk script with phrases such as "I am strong," "I am capable," and "I've got this." Use those mantras to drown out the negative thoughts that pipe up.

TRY SOMETHING NEW: If you've been doing the same sport your whole life, or most of your adult life, it might be time to step away for a brief respite and try something new, even if it's just a different variation on the same sport. For instance, Selene was an elite-level competitive mountain biker for nearly ten years, from her late thirties to her midforties. As she reached her later forties, she found it impossible to compete at the level she was used to. After a year or two of struggling with negative self-talk and constantly comparing herself to her younger self, she simply decided to do something different. She started trail-running, took up stand-up paddle boarding, joined a CrossFit gym, and did more yoga. The change helped her broaden her definition of herself and gave her new challenges to try rather than struggling to repeat the same performances. When she was ready to race again, she switched to gravel and found a renewed passion for the sport; she even managed to stand on a few podiums again. Sometimes a break is all you need to get your motivation and mojo back—or find it again, but for something fresh and new.

GO BACK TO BASICS OR AHEAD TO A MASTER CLASS: Many of us reach a certain point in our favorite sports and activities and we stay there for years . . . maybe decades. That leads to stagnation at best, backsliding at worst. The good news is that now you're perfectly positioned to make gains by taking your form and technique to the next level. If you've been a runner for years, incorporate movement drills, like strides, high knees, and bounding drills, into your repertoire. These form drills open up the communication between your brain and your muscles to improve your coordination, proprioception, and balance, and that makes you a more efficient, faster, and more injury-resistant runner. If you're a swimmer, take some time to master your weakest stroke. Book a few sessions with a trainer to learn some new lifts. Developing more mastery of what you love to do is a surefire way to boost your confidence. And no, you're not too old to learn new things. You never are. Research on adults ranging in age from their fifties to their seventies shows that, with proper instruction, older women and men can learn just as well as those 30 years younger.

DRESS FOR SUCCESS: You've probably read that advice countless times over the years. That's because putting your best foot forward makes a positive impact, even in the context of working out or competing. Having worked numerous "before-and-after" photo shoots for glossy magazines over the years, Selene can tell you that often the women featured haven't lost that much weight or changed their body composition that much. They appear radically different because of the "after" clothing style, not because of any change in their size. For the "before" shots, stylists put them in baggy T-shirts and poorly fitting sweatpants, clothes that make them look shapeless. Most of these women don't smile for the photos because they don't feel attractive. Then the stylists dress them up in fitted, fun clothes that show their shape for the "after" shots. The smiles you see are genuine. The women feel better because they look their best. Clothes that fit well and make you feel good can be transformative. And today there are more companies than ever like Athleta and Machines for Freedom that are making super-flattering workout clothes for women of every size.

FOLLOW INSPIRATIONAL LEADS: Cindy Crawford once famously said, "I wish I looked like Cindy Crawford," alluding to the fact that models are often Photoshopped and airbrushed to the point that they barely recognize themselves. Well, today's photo app tools like Facetune let everyone edit, enhance, and retouch their selfies to the point where they don't look like their real selves. Following these types of "fitspiration" or "fitspo" trainers will not leave you feeling inspired. Better to follow real athletes and active women who focus and showcase what fit, healthy bodies can do at every size. That's real fitspiration.

16

KEEP YOUR SKELETON STRONG

Be good to your bones. They're your foundation.

The statistics are sobering: approximately one in two women over age 50 will break a bone because of osteoporosis. In fact, a woman's risk of breaking a hip is equal to the combined risk of breast, uterine, and ovarian cancer, according to the National Osteoporosis Foundation (NOF).

As mentioned in chapter 7 on plyometrics, menopause is a precarious time for bone health: you can lose one-fifth of your bone density during the five to seven years following menopause. That makes building a strong skeleton priority number one during this time of life.

YOUR LIVING SKELETON

We often think of our bones as solid, inert structures, like the metal girders supporting skyscrapers. But in fact, your bones are constantly remodeling. Mature bone is removed from your skeleton and new bone tissue is formed throughout your life. That's how bones heal when you break them and how you can build stronger bones through the stress of exercise. When you stress your skeleton—for instance, by doing the jumping exercises detailed in chapter 7—you create micro-damage to your bones, which your body repairs and builds back stronger. It's a lot like how strength training for your muscles works.

When you're growing as a kid, this bone-building process is rapid and yields positive gains. One hundred percent of your skeleton is replaced during your first year of life. But then the remodeling efforts decline with age, with only about 10 percent of our skeleton being replaced during early adulthood, according to Duke Orthopaedics. By 30, most of us will have hit peak bone mass, then we experience relatively small declines until the menopause transition, when we start to slide more dramatically in the other direction, according to the NIH Osteoporosis and Related Bone Diseases National Resource Center.

As mentioned in chapter 3, estrogen plays an important role in bone remodeling, so it helps keep the decline in check. With age, everyone, both men and women, loses about 0.5 percent of their bone mass per year.

In women, when sex hormones flatline after menopause and the protective effects of estrogen disappear, bone loss can accelerate to 2 percent annually until it slows to about 1 to 1.5 percent of loss per year a few years postmenopause.

Whether you're just entering perimenopause or have made it all the way to the other side, the sooner you act, the stronger you can make your skeleton and the likelier you are to be able to maintain it. It's especially important to act immediately if you've ever been amenorrheic (stopped menstruating because of relative energy deficiency in sport—RED-S). Amenorrhea causes bone loss during the peak years of building and maintaining bone by causing estrogen levels to drop and remain low. Prolonged RED-S and amenorrhea can cause irreversible bone loss, particularly in the spine. Research suggests, however, that even amenorrheic athletes with diminished bone density can bounce back by their thirties, so long as they recover their estrogen levels and menstrual cycle with adequate nutrition.

START WITH A SCAN

The only way to know the state of your bone health is to get a bone density test, otherwise known as a dual-energy X-ray absorptiometry (DEXA) scan, or DXA scan. The test estimates the density of your bones and your chances of breaking a bone.

NOF recommends that you have a bone density test if:

- *You're a woman age 65 or older*
- *You break a bone after age 50*
- *You are a woman of menopausal age with risk factors for low bone density (see the box, "What's Your Risk?")*
- *You are a postmenopausal woman under age 65 with risk factors*

You should also consider a DEXA scan if:

- *An X-ray of your spine has shown a break or bone loss in your spine*
- *You have back pain with a possible break in your spine*
- *You've lost half an inch or more of height within one year*
- *You've lost one and a half inches or more of your original height*

If you're postmenopausal or over the age of 50, you'll get a T-score, which is a measure of your bone mineral density compared to a young adult.

T-scores of -1.0 and above are considered normal.

T-scores of -1.1 to -2.4 are considered an indication of low bone mass, or osteopenia.

T-scores of -2.5 and lower are considered an indication of osteoporosis.

The lower your T-score, the lower your bone density.

If you're premenopausal or younger than 50, you'll get a Z-score, which is a measure of your bone mineral density compared with others of your gender, ethnicity, and age.

A Z-score of -2.0 is considered below the normal range for your age group.

Being diagnosed with low bone density (also known as osteopenia) does not mean you are destined to get osteoporosis, but it does give you a greater chance of developing the disease if you lose too much bone in the future.

As mentioned in chapter 7, if you're diagnosed with osteoporosis, you should talk with your health care provider about what exercise is safe (or not safe) for you. You may need to avoid high-impact exercises such as jumping and running, as well as exercises that involve a lot of bending (like abdominal crunches, which aren't very useful anyway) and twisting (like golf), as they put too much pressure on the vertebrae of your spine. But you definitely want to perform resistance training two to three days a week.

BUILD YOUR BONES

Your skeleton supports you and your muscles put you in motion. So every move you make is the product of your muscles pulling on your bones to take you in the direction you want to go. The more those movements stress your skeleton, the more your body responds by making your bones denser and stronger.

Regular exercise can prevent bone loss and replace some lost bone when you're older. The best activities for promoting bone remodeling are the ones that force your body to work against gravity, also known as weight-bearing activities, and those that create a little impact, which further stimulates your skeleton. Sports like walking, running, dancing, and tennis are good bone-builders. Swimming and cycling, which are low-impact and non-weight-bearing, are helpful, because they put some strain on the muscle, but you need that additional impact for optimum skeletal health.

Strength training is also an excellent bone-builder. Postmenopausal women with low and even very low bone density see significant bone density gains—improving about 1 percent per year—in their spine and hips, two of the areas most susceptible to osteoporosis, when they participate in a regular strength training program.

Pay special attention to posture exercises, such as moves for your upper back that strengthen the muscles between your shoulder blades. These can strengthen your spine-supporting muscles and reduce the sloping shoulders and rounding-forward posture that older women can get as they lose muscle mass and strength. This condition, called kyphosis, can be the result of bad posture as well as compression fractures in the spine. Keeping your upper back muscles strong can help prevent both.

Women who have been diagnosed with osteoporosis can—and should—still lift heavy sh*t. Research shows that high-intensity weight training is better for your thinning bones than lower-intensity training.

In the 2017 "LiftMOR" study published in the *Journal of Bone and Mineral Research*, researchers took a group of 101 women whose average age was 65 (all were at least 58) and who had been diagnosed with low bone density. After a month of foundation training, the researchers had them either lift heavy sh*t or do low-intensity lifting. The heavy lifters did a supervised program of deadlifts, overhead presses, and back squats, performing five sets of five repetitions twice a week. This group also added some impact by doing jumping chin-ups with drop landings. The lower-intensity group performed a home-based program that included 10 to 15 reps of exercises like lunges, calf raises, and shrugs twice a week. They also performed a general stretching routine.

After eight months, the high-intensity lifters experienced consistently superior improvements in bone mineral density in the hip and lumbar spine area. Fewer high-intensity lifters than low-intensity lifters saw a decline in bone mineral density. The heavy lifters also enjoyed the most improvements in functional performance tests. None of the heavy lifters experienced injuries, beyond one minor low-back muscle strain that limited training for a week.

That said, it's *especially* important, if you're a woman with low bone density, to get proper exercise instruction and supervision from a knowledgeable professional. It's important to perform these exercises with proper form and intensity, so that you're placing the load where you want it and not where you don't.

BONE-BUILDING FOODS

The National Dairy Council has successfully made milk nearly synonymous with bone health. But that connection is tenuous at best. The 12-year Nurses' Health Study, which included more than 77,000 registered nurses, reported that women who drank a lot of milk—two or more glasses per day—were no less likely to break a hip than their peers who drank it once a week. The same was true for higher intakes of calcium from other foods.

That's not to say you don't need calcium, a mineral that is a key ingredient for building bones. Nearly all your body's calcium is stored in your bones and teeth, where it supports their structure and hardness. Your body also uses calcium to regulate your heart rhythm, transmit nerve impulses to contract your muscles, and help your blood clot. When you don't have enough, your body dips into your bones (the body's calcium bank) to take what it needs. So sufficient calcium is important. Research is still a bit equivocal on exactly how much and what the best sources are. Currently the Institute of Medicine calls for women over 50 to get 1,200 milligrams a day and for those under 50 to get 1,000 milligrams a day.

You also need vitamin D, which plays a critical role in maintaining bone health, as well as vitamin K, which is an underappreciated nutrient. Low levels of vitamin K have been linked to low bone density. The Nurses' Health Study found that eating at least 100 micrograms of vitamin K a day (there are about 50 in a cup of lettuce and 220 in a cup of broccoli) can slash your risk of hip fracture by 30 percent.

Magnesium is looking increasingly important as well. A 2020 study published in *Maturitas* listed magnesium, along with vitamin K2 (which is found in cheese, egg yolk, and fermented foods), vitamin D, and calcium, as key to the management of osteoporosis. High-magnesium foods include dark leafy greens, nuts, seeds, avocados, beans, and fish.

Getting all these nutrients together in your daily diet is the best strategy for building a strong skeleton. Reach for fatty fish like sardines and salmon, which have even more vitamin D than milk. Certain yogurts are fortified with calcium and vitamin D. And broccoli, Brussels sprouts, kale, and other dark leafy greens (which are also excellent for microbiome and hormonal health) will deliver vitamin K as well as calcium and magnesium.

Foods like olive oil, soy beans, blueberries and foods rich in omega-3s (like fatty fish) may also have bone-building benefits, according to the National Osteoporosis Foundation.

Some women may need to supplement their diet for optimum bone health. You can learn more about supplements in chapter 18.

BAD TO THE BONE

Just as some foods and lifestyle habits like exercise can fortify your bones, others can rob your bone banks of the precious minerals they need to stay strong. Two big ones that are likely not an issue if you're reading these words right now are smoking and being sedentary, both of which raise your risk for osteoporosis.

Alcohol use appears to go either way, depending on if you use it wisely and in moderation. Some epidemiological studies have linked moderate intake of alcohol with decreased fracture risk in postmenopausal women. This is certainly not a reason to drink, however, because animal studies show no benefit of alcohol to bones (so there are likely other factors at work) and there's no question that heavy drinking is bad for them. If you do drink, stick to one drink (12 ounces of beer, 5 ounces of wine, or 1.5 ounces of spirits) a day.

Though some experts used to believe that caffeine use could be bad for skeletal health, the Hong Kong Osteoporosis Study published in 2020 found the opposite: people who habitually drank coffee had higher bone mass density than non-coffee drinkers.

There is evidence that too much soda can weaken your bones by altering your body's balance of calcium and phosphorus in an unfavorable direction. The Framingham Osteoporosis Study found that women who reported drinking cola every day had lower bone density than women who reported drinking it less than once a month. More recently, a 2020 study of more than 17,000 adults published in *Nutrients* found that soft drink consumption was directly associated with the risk of fracture and that daily consumption of soft drinks was associated with a doubled risk of fractures. Soda and sugary soft drinks aren't really good for you, so if bone health is a concern, this is an easy place to make a positive change.

Finally, keep your stress levels in check. (See chapter 15 for plenty of stress-busting strategies.) In a 2019 study of more than 11,000 postmenopausal women over a period of six years, researchers found that high amounts of social stress— such as the stress that comes from relationships and other social interactions— was associated with lower bone mineral density, even after researchers accounted for age at menopause, chronic health problems, smoking, alcohol use, hormone therapy, physical activity, weight, and history of fractures.

WHAT'S YOUR RISK?

Simply being a female (especially a menopausal or postmenopausal one) puts you at a higher risk for osteoporosis: women comprise 80 percent of the people with the disease in the United States. But there are myriad other factors to keep in mind, according to the

Bone Health & Osteoporosis Foundation. Here's what raises your risk:

Being of Asian or Caucasian ethnicity

Long-term use of oral glucocorticoid medication (prednisone)

Being sedentary

Having a small frame

Smoking

Alcohol use of more than two drinks per day

Family history of osteoporosis

History of unresolved amenorrhea

Having hyperparathyroidism

Having bowel diseases (because of poor nutrient absorption)

17

STRATEGIES FOR EXERCISING THROUGH THE TRANSITION

You don't have to let menopause symptoms send you to the sidelines.

In triathlons, the transition between sports is often referred to as the "third sport," because it takes strategy and practice to get from the swim to the bike to the run quickly and seamlessly. Well, you can think of managing your menopausal symptoms as the "fourth sport." (Lucky us! We get another sport!)

Seriously. Anyone who has ever tried to negotiate hot flashes, heavy periods, achy joints, and the like knows that the struggle is *real*. But none of it is insurmountable. Here we take a look at how to navigate your symptoms while maintaining your active life through the menopausal transition.

HOT FLASHES

If only we could time our hot flashes to when we could actually use them—like when we're putting in freezing cold base miles on our bikes in the dead of winter. Sadly, no one has figured out an app for that yet, so we need to deal with hot flashes when they come—often at the most inopportune times!

Though exercise is obviously good for your overall health and well-being and helps you maintain a healthy weight, which is linked to a lower incidence of hot flashes, it does not prevent hot flashes per se. Some research shows that being physically active enables you to have fewer hot flashes, but other research shows that they may be more severe. A study published in the *American Journal of Human Biology* found that women who reported performing at higher levels of physical activity were at significantly higher risk of having moderate to severe hot flashes, though they were not at risk of having more hot flashes overall. Body composition plays a major role here, regardless of exercise. Higher body fat increases the risk of more severe hot flashes; the likelihood of developing vasomotor symptoms like hot flashes decreases significantly as lean body mass increases, according to a 2020 study published in *Women's Midlife Health* that pulled data from 2,533 women who were part of the Study of Women's Health Across the Nation (SWAN).

Blame declining estrogen levels. When you're premenopausal, your blood vessels expand as you warm up, sending blood closer to your skin to help you cool off. Estrogen assists with that process. Later, when your estrogen levels are in decline, that response is blunted and you end up with more heat trapped in your core. Recall, too, that the body's thermostat is more likely to overreact to changes in temperature because (again) your hormones aren't there to help regulate it. The result: hot flashes.

There's no inherent health risk to training through hot flashes, but they can certainly be annoying and disruptive. Having ice-cold hydration on hand can help create a heat sink and cool you from the inside. I also recommend cooling your skin at key points of your body, like the back of your neck. Cyclists often make cooling socks by filling pantyhose full of ice and knotting them at both ends; they slip these down the back of their jersey to stay cooler. Runners can try products like Kafka Kool Ties, which are lightweight scarfs filled with cooling beads, to get the same effect.

Layering is key. Hot flashes often cause you to swing from overheated to chilled in whiplash fashion. Having a lightweight jacket or vest that you can zip and unzip to let off steam or trap heat as needed can go a long way.

Also be sure to stay well hydrated in general to help with your temperature control (see chapter 12).

ERRATIC PERIODS AND PMS

Menopause means the end of your period as you know it, but your menstrual cycle is not going "gentle into that good night," as the poet said. For many women, it's quite the opposite: their periods—and their PMS—seem to go into temporary overdrive.

If this happens to you and becomes unmanageably disruptive, do not hesitate to talk to your health care provider about MHT. It can be a lifesaver for erratic periods, heavy bleeding, and raging PMS symptoms. As mentioned previously, often an IUD or progestin-only pills can even out your hormones and make this transition more manageable.

If you've read *ROAR*, you know there are some tricks to help you work with your menstrual cycle swings. Here's a little redux for managing them as you approach menopause:

TIME YOUR CARB INTAKE: You burn more calories overall during your premenstrual period, but even though you are more sensitive to carbs during menopause, you still need them in your system if you're doing long bouts of intense exercise. Aim for a combination of 10 to 15 grams of protein and 40 grams of carbs (about 200 to 220 calories) before any workout longer than 90 minutes, and 40 to 50 grams of carbs with protein and fat (through real food) per hour during long workouts.

CURB THE CRAMPS: Yep, cramps can and do still happen. If you track your cycle via apps like Wild.AI, you can head them off at the pass by taking magnesium, omega-3 fatty acids, and a low-dose 80-milligram aspirin in the week leading up to your period. Aspirin suppresses the production of prostaglandin-E2 (the prostaglandin associated with the menstrual cycle), which reduces the effect of these cramp-causing chemicals. Your body uses more magnesium for building the endometrial lining, so it pulls magnesium from other cellular functions, like muscle contractions. If you're low in magnesium, you'll have ineffective muscle contractions and spasms—akin to a muscle cramp during exercise—when the uterus contracts. Omega-3s counter the prostaglandins as well. For the best result, take 200 milligrams of magnesium and 1 gram of omega-3.

DO A GUT CHECK: The same prostaglandins that cause cramps can trigger other smooth muscles, like the ones in your bowels, to react similarly, leaving you with diarrhea or loose stools, gas, and painful gut spasms. Following the same anti-cramping strategies just mentioned can help. Also, be sure to heed the advice in chapter 8 on maintaining gut health. The unchecked stress hormones and elevated inflammation common at this time can cause imbalances in the gut microbiome, exacerbating any GI distress you're already experiencing. Fermented foods like kimchi, kefir, and yogurt should be a daily staple in a perimenopausal athlete's diet.

STEM THE FLOW: Heavy periods happen. And during perimenopause, they can happen when you least expect them. Keep a stash of products any and every place you might need them—your gym bag, your glove compartment, your office—so that you don't need to sit out a workout for fear of having a mess on your hands (and legs).

Menstrual cups, which are small flexible cups you insert in your vagina during your period, can be a godsend for heavy bleeding because they are less likely to leak and easier to just empty and reinsert when you need to rather than burning through multiple tampons or trying to manage pads.

When you're cycling, your chamois will be there to protect you should leakage occur. For other activities, you can invest in a pair of "period underwear," like Thinx or Knix; these highly absorbent undergarments are specifically made for wearing during menstruation.

HEAD OFF HEADACHES

As mentioned in chapter 3, as your hormone levels shift you can end up with perimenopausal headaches, even if you've never been prone to headaches before. If you were prone to PMS-related headaches, they can get worse before they get better once your hormone fluctuations die down. Headaches are generally brought on by a change in blood pressure and sudden dilation and constriction of your blood vessels, along with a decline in serotonin levels (which helps the communication between nerve cells and is involved in the pain-sensing process).

For some women, headache frequency ramps up significantly during perimenopause. That's clearly not conducive to being on your A-game. Staying hydrated helps by maintaining healthy circulation. Foods rich in nitrates convert to nitric oxide (NO) in the body, so eating more of these foods will widen your blood vessels, reducing the severity of headache during the perimenopausal shift. Nitrate-rich foods include beets, pomegranate, watermelon, and spinach. MHT is a mixed bag. Research shows it can improve, worsen, or make no changes in headaches depending on the type of hormone therapy you use and the type of headaches you get.

BEAT THE BLAHS

Some women just feel "meh" during their menopausal years, as though their spark was snuffed out and their mojo is stuck on low. Managing stress, which we talked about in chapter 15, is a biggie here, especially when you're experiencing mood swings and MIA motivation. Increasing your circulating amino acids can also help. If you haven't already upped your BCAA intake for your muscles, do it for your moods.

As you know, hormones affect different regions of your brain. Estrogen and progesterone affect the hypothalamus, which helps regulate fatigue and emotional control and is interconnected with the central nervous system. As your hormones fluctuate and decline, you can find yourself pushing through—literally—fatigue, lethargy, and low mood. Estrogen also increases serotonin, an excess of which can impair central nervous system function, creating mental and physical fatigue. Taking in more BCAAs, especially leucine, can help lift your spirits and reignite (or at least protect) your spark. Leucine crosses the blood-brain barrier, slows down the effect of serotonin, and helps prevent central nervous system fatigue.

VAGINAL PAIN

About half of women develop symptoms from vaginal atrophy—now known as genitourinary syndrome of menopause (GSM), the thinning of the vaginal tissues due to loss of estrogen. A dry, itchy vagina can put a huge damper on your sex life. That alone is obvious—and something to definitely address—but it also can make exercise like bike riding and even running painful. Some cyclists start using extra chamois cream, applied very liberally to their labia. But that's just (literally) masking the problem.

Other options actually help rebuild atrophying vaginal tissues and bring natural moisture back, so exercise (and sex) are not painful. There are two prescription options:

VAGINAL ESTROGEN: Vaginal estrogen, which comes in creams, tablets (that you insert), and estrogen-infused vaginal rings, works to thicken thinning vaginal walls and restore mucosal cells. The nice thing about vaginal estrogen is that the doses are very low and localized, so it's safe even for women who don't want to or can't take oral estrogen. According to the American College of Obstetricians and Gynecologists (ACOG), using it does not increase the chance of breast cancer or the chance of a recurrence in those who have a history of the disease. Vaginal estrogen also helps relieve other disruptive symptoms like urinary incontinence and frequent vaginal infections and urinary tract infections (UTIs).

VAGINAL DHEA: Your body uses dehydroepiandrosterone (DHEA) to produce estrogens and androgens (like testosterone). Used topically, it can improve vaginal tissue and moisture. Like vaginal estrogen, it doesn't produce any systemic effects.

The best nonprescription options are Replens Long-Lasting Vaginal Moisturizer and Revaree Vaginal Moisturizer. These are good alternatives for women who don't want to use prescription products like estrogen or DHEA. They work by drawing moisture into the vaginal lining. Each application lasts up to three days, so you don't have to use it every day. They are also FDA-approved.

INCONTINENCE

Nearly half of women over 50 say that they sometimes leak urine (urinary incontinence), according to a poll by the University of Michigan Institute for Policy and Innovation. Up to 20 percent of women stop running and doing other exercise because they wet themselves, according to the National Association for Continence. Giving up exercise because of urinary incontinence is completely unnecessary. The core work and breathing exercises detailed in chapter 14 can help mitigate the urinary incontinence that often occurs during the menopausal years. The advice for vaginal dryness and atrophy can also help here. If you try those remedies and still get no relief, see a pelvic floor specialist. This is a condition that is largely treatable.

While you are working on stopping the leaks, you can stay in the game by using some strategies that will help you avoid embarrassing wetness while you work out.

AVOID BLADDER IRRITANTS: Caffeine and spicy foods can cause bladder irritation in some people. If you consume a lot of either or both, try dialing back and see if that helps.

WEAR PROTECTION: You can wear light incontinence pads for small leaks. Also, brands like Thinx and Fancypants sell protective "pee-proof" underwear (similar to those for menstruation).

BODY ODOR

I'm putting this one in here so you'll know it's not your imagination if you've noticed that your body odor is stronger than it used to be. There are several reasons: You're likely sweating more because of hot flashes and night sweats. You also may be more stressed out, and that produces more sweat from your apocrine glands—a thick, fatty type of sweat that bacteria feeds on, creating an unpleasant odor. Hormonal changes and changes in the bacteria on your skin also contribute to more unpleasant body odors. You may need to switch to a stronger antiperspirant or deodorant.

DOMS AND ACHES

Unchecked inflammation and impaired protein synthesis (the process that helps repair and make new muscle tissue) can leave you vulnerable to higher levels of muscle soreness like delayed onset muscle soreness (DOMS) following a hard workout.

Your first line of defense is making sure that you have enough protein and key amino acids coursing through your circulation before and after your workouts to keep from getting catabolic (eating your own muscle tissue) and to jump-start repair when you're done. A 2019 meta-analysis of the effect of BCAA supplementation and muscle soreness following exercise showed that "a large decrease in DOMS occurs following BCAA supplementation after exercise compared to a placebo [dummy pill] supplement."

Again, the BCAA leucine appears to be a key player here, as animal research shows that leucine-enriched amino acids (LEAA) improve the rate of muscle protein synthesis and lessen the muscle soreness generally associated with DOMS.

Reducing inflammation will also help you avoid being sidelined with muscle soreness. A diet rich in anti-inflammatory foods is key. Choose foods that are rich in the natural inflammation-fighting omega-3 fatty acids such as mackerel, salmon, tuna, and other fatty fish. Also rich in natural anti-inflammatories are berries and fruits like blackberries, blueberries, watermelon, and cherries; leafy greens like spinach, kale, and collards; olive oil; and nuts like almonds and walnuts. Avoid inflammatory foods like fried foods, sugary sodas, refined carbs, and processed meats.

The Indian spice curcumin may also help with inflammation and muscle soreness, according to a 2015 study published in the *European Journal of Applied Physiology*, which reported that curcumin supplementation "likely reduces pain associated with DOMS with some evidence for enhanced recovery of muscle performance." So curcumin may help reduce pain and increase strength.

And of course, there's always the tried-and-true method: taking a nice hot bath. There are many bath bombs, like those infused with CBD, that promise to increase relaxation and recovery. There's no conclusive science there. But there's no doubt that a hot soak can be just what the doctor ordered for tired, sore muscles.

See "Smart Recovery Practices" in chapter 13 for more ways to avoid DOMS.

POST-EXERCISE WOBBLES AND WOOZINESS

Clients sometimes tell me that they're getting woozy and wobbly in ways they never have before and feel like they suddenly need a fainting couch after hard workouts.

Blame those blood vessel changes. Just as they're slower to expand now when you start working out, they also are slower to shrink back to normal, sedentary size. This can cause a sudden blood pressure drop that leaves you light-headed when you stop exercising. (It's also why you may feel like the world is swimming when you stand up too fast.)

Even if you've always been one of those women who just stops in her tracks after the last interval, now is the time to take a minute or two for a proper cool-down to let your body change gears. Drinking a cold recovery drink can speed up the process. It also helps to work out in compression wear, which keeps the blood moving back up from your lower extremities instead of pooling in your legs.

KEEP MOVING

Many menopausal athletes tell me that, though they feel like they need more recovery time now, they don't do very well when they are completely sedentary for a full day, because everything seems to get more stiff and sore.

Movement is medicine for your muscles! So even on days when you don't have an exercise session scheduled, be sure to include plenty of daily activity like walking the dog, doing a little gardening, or whatever you like to do that keeps your body moving.

Movement is important for your overall health too. Studies show that even if you exercise regularly, being sedentary the majority of the time wreaks havoc on your health. One study published in the February 2021 issue of *Medicine & Science in Sports & Exercise* reported that even if you regularly exercise, if you're otherwise sedentary, taking just 2,500 to 5,000 steps a day, you can actually develop "exercise resistance," meaning that your fat-burning abilities are impaired by your general inactivity. That means that prolonged sitting and inactivity can wash out the benefits you get from exercising. So keep moving!

18

SUPPLEMENTS: WHAT YOU NEED AND WHAT YOU DON'T

Health and performance can sometimes be helped with a pill.

I'm obviously very open to supporting one's body through supplements. The adaptogens that I recommend and use (see chapter 4) are a prime example of well-appointed supplements that can improve your quality of life, especially during menopause, when your physiology is fluctuating and changing rather quickly and dramatically.

However, there can be a tendency to overdo pills and powders and potions. Some women's kitchen cabinets resemble a CVS pharmacy, they're so packed with bottles and bags. Somewhat ironically, healthy, active people are the biggest consumers of these products because we have a keen desire to stay healthy as well as boost our performance, quicken recovery, and of course stave off disease. We're also more likely to seek out natural solutions to make us healthier and stronger.

But our desire to boost our health and performance also makes us susceptible to a lot of product promises that may be high on hype but rather thin on science. So, while a few supplements undoubtedly may actually improve your performance and general health, most are a waste of money and may even be detrimental. Supplements are also largely unregulated. The FDA doesn't oversee their quality, and when independent watchdogs like *Consumer Reports* dig in, they often find that many of the products they test don't really contain what's listed on the label.

So with that in mind, I always encourage women to tread very carefully when they're wading into these waters. My underlying philosophy is that you should work with your own physiology to become the best you can be. What I like about adaptogens is that they do just that. Any other vitamins, minerals, or phytonutrients you consider taking should be shown to provide the same benefits.

Obviously, science has evolved since then, and menopausal women have very specific needs. So here is an updated and expanded version of supplement facts just for you.

VITAMINS AND MINERALS

Vitamins and minerals are nearly always best obtained through foods and natural sources rather than in pill or capsule form. There are some exceptions, but often women can do more harm than good by taking too many of these supplements. We touched upon some of these in *ROAR*. This updated and expanded list covers the vitamins and minerals that affect you most during this time of life.

VITAMIN D: Vitamin D, also called the "sunshine vitamin," plays a prominent role in our health, wellness, and performance, especially as we get older. It's unique in that it is both a nutrient we get from food and a hormone that our bodies make.

The fat-soluble vitamin helps the body absorb and retain calcium and phosphorus, so it's critical for bone health. Maintaining bone health isn't only a woman's issue, but it does tend to be a more urgent issue for women: 80 percent of the 10 million Americans with osteoporosis are female, and one in two women over the age of 50 will break a bone because of osteoporosis in her lifetime. (See chapter 16 for more information on bone health.)

Vitamin D is also essential for immune function, heart health, and muscle function. It can be tricky to get this vitamin from food unless you eat a lot of fatty fish like salmon, tuna, and mackerel. Fortified milk, cheese, and egg yolks also contain vitamin D, but the primary source for most humans is the sun, which reacts with our skin to synthesize the essential nutrient.

It turns out that many of us aren't getting enough vitamin D from any source. In fact, some researchers have gone so far as to call vitamin D deficiency a pandemic (a word none of us want to hear again after 2020!). Some experts believe that we lack vitamin D because we spend so much of our modern lives indoors, and when we do go out, we cover ourselves in clothes and sunblock. The sunblock part is iffy. Some studies have found that sunblock can indeed hinder vitamin D synthesis from sunshine. Others have found the effect negligible. One study based in Australia found no differences in vitamin D levels between people who were assigned to use sunscreen one summer and those assigned a placebo cream.

Other factors play a role too. People with darker skin require more UVB exposure than light-skinned people to generate the same amounts of vitamin D. Older adults are not able to convert UVB light into vitamin D as readily as younger adults. And the farther you live from the equator, the less vitamin D–producing UVB rays you'll be exposed to, especially during the winter.

Ultimately, you don't need to spread out a blanket and deliberately bake yourself with baby oil like it's 1986, but we can't ignore the problem either because vitamin D is a key player in many essential metabolic functions. This is especially true for menopausal women: estrogen plays a role in activating vitamin D, and so declining estrogen levels can worsen vitamin D deficiency at this time of life.

You can get your vitamin D levels checked via a simple blood test. Vitamin D levels of 50 nanomoles per liter (nmol/L) are considered sufficient, although the Endocrine Society argues that your levels should be more than 75 nmol/L to maximize the effect of vitamin D on calcium, bone, and muscle metabolism.

Increasing your vitamin D levels (especially if they are low) may help with physical performance on nearly every level. In fact, research indicates that maintaining your vitamin D levels at 75 to 100 nmol/L could boost your aerobic capacity, muscle growth, and muscle power, shorten your recovery time from hard exercise bouts, and improve bone density. More than that, however, is not better. Very high levels of vitamin D (more than 125 nmol/L) can have negative side effects.

You can stay safe by keeping your supplementation below 4,000 IUs of vitamin D.

IRON: Your body uses iron, an essential mineral, to build the red blood cells that carry fresh oxygen to your muscles via your bloodstream. When your levels are low, you run the risk of iron-deficiency anemia, which can leave you chronically tired, hamper your workouts, and also cause more random symptoms like being irritable and frequently feeling cold.

Iron deficiency is a more common diagnosis in women than in men, owing to the even greater iron loss women experience through red cell breakdown, losses in sweat, gastrointestinal bleeding (from running impact, gut distress, and NSAID use), and an increase in cytokine expression (inflammation by-products that interfere with the absorption of iron) from the constant acute inflammation response to exercise.

Taking an iron supplement often improves exercise performance in *premenopausal* woman. A meta-analysis of iron supplements and exercise performance in women of reproductive age done by Australian researchers found that female athletes (particularly those low in iron) who took iron supplements improved their maximum power as well as their exercise efficiency—that is, they put out more power at a lower heart rate.

However, getting the dosing right can be tricky, because oral supplements impact your hepcidin levels; hepcidin regulates iron metabolism, and high hepcidin levels reduce your gut's ability to absorb iron. A 2020 study published in the journal *Haematologica* reported that in iron-depleted women without anemia, iron supplements increased levels of hepcidin for 24 hours, which decreased the absorption of supplements taken the next day. The researchers concluded that iron might be most effectively absorbed if taken every other day. (They couldn't say for sure if this would be the case for women with full-blown anemia.) Your menstrual cycle (for perimenopausal women) may also impact your body's ability to absorb iron.

For perimenopausal women, the story is further complicated by estrogen fluctuations. During this time, as you'll recall, you can find yourself with relatively high levels of estrogen, which can lead to systemic inflammation. That inflammation in turn increases levels of hepcidin. Again, when hepcidin is too high, your iron levels can become too low, leaving you with iron deficiency and the fatigue characteristic of anemia. Taking an iron supplement won't help because the hepcidin reduces the absorption. So what to do?

We know that taking vitamin D suppresses hepcidin expression, and that it also promotes erythropoiesis (making red blood cells). So being sure that you're getting enough vitamin D as mentioned earlier is the first step.

Postmenopause, your iron needs change, as you're not losing blood every month. That's why the USDA recommends that women ages 19 to 50 need at least 18 milligrams of iron a day, but that after age 50 the need for iron drops down to just 8 milligrams a day. Research shows that as estrogen decreases by 90 percent during the transition from premenopause to postmenopause, iron levels increase two- to threefold. But the story is complicated for active women. Research shows that hepcidin levels in postmenopausal women who do high-intensity exercise stay elevated for up to 24 hours, reducing all iron metabolism. This is why newly postmenopausal women are susceptible to iron deficiency.

The general rule is to just eat a healthy diet and get your iron that way. Iron is easy to get, especially if you eat meat, poultry, or seafood, which are all good sources of heme iron. Heme iron is easier for the body to absorb than the non-heme iron in plant sources. To maximize the amount of iron your body absorbs, eat iron-rich foods with foods rich in vitamin C, such as citrus, peppers, leafy greens, and tomatoes. Vitamin C is particularly important for vegetarians and vegans because it helps increase the absorption of iron from plant foods.

Generally speaking, every woman should consider getting her iron levels checked through a routine blood screening, especially if they're feeling fatigued or not as strong and energetic as usual during their workouts. If you train and race, it could be worth getting screened even if you feel normal, because you could be low in iron and not know it. At that point, your doctor can work with you on a supplementation plan that includes follow-ups.

MAGNESIUM: Magnesium is an essential mineral that your body uses to maintain healthy blood pressure and muscle and nerve function, regulate blood sugar, build bone, and more. Magnesium is easy to obtain through a healthy diet, as it is widely distributed in a variety of plant and animal foods, including green leafy vegetables, legumes, nuts, seeds, and whole grains, as well as fish, poultry, and beef.

Still, suboptimal magnesium status is common among people in the United States, with nearly half of us not getting what we need in our diet. Your risk for having lower magnesium levels increases with your activity levels. When you exercise strenuously, you pee and sweat out enough magnesium to increase your magnesium requirement by up to 20 percent, according to research.

In other words, if you routinely get the 320 milligrams recommended each day for adult women, you could easily be deficient if you're very active. This is a concern since research shows that maintaining healthy magnesium levels is especially important for maintaining muscle and preventing muscle loss in women as they age. Getting enough magnesium can also help reduce some of the most common menopause symptoms, including poor sleep, mood swings, anxiety, and a heightened risk of heart disease.

If you're highly active or could use help alleviating your menopausal symptoms, consider taking a magnesium supplement to keep your levels in the recommended range.

CALCIUM: Women have been pushed and prompted to take calcium as a preventative measure against osteoporosis for decades. And you know what? As we mentioned in chapter 16, it might be a wash. At best, the science is very inconclusive.

In 2013, the United States Preventive Services Task Force recommended that postmenopausal women refrain from taking calcium. After reviewing more than 135 studies, the task force concluded that calcium supplementation didn't prevent fractures. Worse, some research suggested that calcium supplements seemed to increase the risk of heart attack.

In contrast, a few large studies, like the Women's Health Initiative, have reported benefits, specifically a reduction in hip fracture among postmenopausal women on hormone therapy taking 1,000 milligrams of calcium and 400 international units of vitamin D a day. (The hormone therapy is a key player here.) And the National Osteoporosis Foundation still recommends supplement use for women with osteoporosis or significant risk factors for a fracture. It's important to note, however, that this is the recommendation for women who are low in calcium to begin with. Too much calcium supplementation, especially when you're getting what you need from your diet, is what appears to be problematic.

Generally speaking, it is wise to err on the side of common sense and get the calcium you need through your diet, not a pill. Some scientists speculate that it's the pills—not the nutrient itself—that may cause the heart problems in some people. When you take a huge bolus of calcium, it just gets dumped into your bloodstream all at once, creating calcium deposits in your arteries; that doesn't happen with the smaller doses you get throughout the day through your diet.

If you're younger than 50, you need 1,000 milligrams a day. Women over 50 need 1,200 milligrams a day. Getting those amounts through food alone is fairly easy. Three servings of plain yogurt (415 milligrams per 8 ounces) can help you get there quickly. One and a half ounces of part skim mozzarella and 3 ounces of sardines both deliver about 330 to 325 milligrams of calcium (33 percent of your daily recommendations). For those who don't eat dairy, fortified cereal and greens such as kale are also good sources. With a calcium-rich diet, no supplementation is necessary.

ANTIOXIDANTS: You do not need, nor should you take, antioxidant supplements. These "superhero" nutrients became extremely popular in the 1990s because of their ability to squash cell-damaging free radicals. But as usual, getting their benefits is not as simple as popping a pill.

As a refresher, antioxidants are molecules that step in and neutralize potentially cell-damaging by-products called free radicals. Free radicals have been blamed for everything from cancer to skin wrinkles, even for aging itself. So looking back, it's not hard to see where our infatuation with antioxidants came from. A tall stack of epidemiological data (large population studies) found that folks who ate a diet filled with antioxidant-rich fruits, vegetables, and drinks had lower rates of disease and lived longer and healthier lives. But when people started taking antioxidant supplements, they didn't get the same effects. They actually got sicker. Two large studies of more than 47,000 smokers taking beta-carotene actually had to be halted because the groups taking the antioxidants were getting both cancer and heart disease at higher rates than those taking dummy pills. The researchers discovered that though foods rich in beta-carotene seemed protective for smokers, one whopping dose of the antioxidant seemed to fortify the free radicals and cause great harm. In fact, *years* after that study was halted, the rates of lung cancer and death among the beta-carotene group were still higher.

So skip the supplements, and while you're at it, check the labels for the sports nutrition foods you're using; some carry hefty doses of these nutrients. If a product is fortified with antioxidants, stop using it. You're doing yourself a disservice. Antioxidants can actually impair your training adaptations and recovery.

We can't outsmart nature. We need to let our bodies naturally overcome exercise-induced stress and make the appropriate adaptations. Look to real food to get everything your body needs for high-level performance and limit supplementation to very specific and medically necessary situations.

Not only do natural foods contain proper amounts of specific nutrients, but they also naturally pair those nutrients with others that work synergistically to provide you with the health benefit. Nowhere is that more true than with antioxidants.

MENOPAUSE AND PERFORMANCE-ENHANCING COMPOUNDS

As long as there have been athletes there have been people trying to use various ergogenic aids—products intended to enhance strength, endurance, stamina, or recovery—to improve their performance. There are also a growing number of supplements targeted specifically at menopausal women. As with vitamins and minerals, most of them are not worth your money. But there are a few standouts:

DI INDOLYL METHANE (DIM): Diindolylmethane is formed in the body from a chemical called indole-3-carbinol, which is found in cruciferous vegetables, which include cabbage, Brussels sprouts, cauliflower, and broccoli. DIM moderates estrogen metabolism by increasing the ratio of favorable estrogen by-products called metabolites to less favorable metabolites. What does that mean? Metabolites are produced when your body breaks down or modifies a molecule or substance. The estrogen hormone can be modified by the addition of one oxygen and hydrogen molecule (OH, a hydroxyl group). Where this group is tacked onto estrogen (which is signified by numbers like 2-OH estrogen or 4-OH estrogen) makes an immense difference in how it acts in your body: some are anti-inflammatory and friendly in the body, while others are associated with inflammation, cell proliferation, and even increases in breast cancer risk.

DIM can help prevent or reverse the estrogen dominance that is common during perimenopause, and it supports hormone balance by encouraging the production of "friendly" estrogen metabolites (2-OH estrogens) with a much gentler, less pronounced estrogenic effect. At the same time, DIM reduces the production of the much more potent, proliferative, and inflammatory estrogens, such as 16-OH estrogens and 4-OH estrogens. The "undesirable" reactive 16-OH estrogen metabolites can exert up to 10 times the level of estrogenic influence as the "friendly" 2-OH metabolites. And the 4-OH variety of metabolite can be really nasty. It can cause what are called DNA adducts, which bind to your genes, raise inflammation, and are associated with uncontrolled mutations and divisions in cells (an increased risk of breast cancer). On the flip side, there is some scientific evidence that DIM may reduce breast cancer risk.

One note of caution: Do *not* take DIM if you're taking estrogen. It will reduce the efficacy.

CREATINE: When I told Selene that we should include creatine in this section, she looked at me quizzically, wondering perhaps whether my love of CrossFit–type training had sent me down the bodybuilding road. Creatine has long been associated with increasing muscle mass, but that is exactly why it might be especially important and beneficial for menopausal women.

Research shows that women have 70 to 80 percent lower creatine stores than men and that we typically consume significantly lower amounts of dietary creatine compared to men. But there hasn't been much research on women and creatine, and some experts have questioned whether or not women athletes would benefit from supplementation.

As it turns out, we can indeed benefit from creatine supplementation. A 2016 study in the *Strength and Conditioning Journal* concluded that women respond to creatine supplementation similarly to men and see increases in both strength and high-intensity type exercises.

A 2021 review of the literature published in *Nutrients* reported that creatine supplementation "may be particularly important during menses, pregnancy, postpartum, during and post-menopause." That's pretty much all women across their life span. The researchers also noted that "females with varying levels of training and fitness may experience improvements in both anaerobic and aerobic exercise performance from both short-term and long-term creatine supplementation."

It may also help with mood disorders. One study found that women with a major depressive disorder who augmented their daily antidepressant with 5 grams of creatine responded twice as fast and experienced remission of depression at twice the rate of women who just took the antidepressant.

For menopausal women specifically, creatine supplementation in combination with resistance training may help counteract muscle, bone, and strength loss by reducing inflammation, oxidative stress, and bone resorption, while also increasing bone formation. The research suggests that taking high doses of creatine (0.3 grams per kilogram a day for at least seven days) may increase muscle mass and function and also improve mood and cognition.

The researchers in the 2021 review recommended a traditional loading dose of 0.3 grams per kilogram of body weight per day for five to seven days, after which you can take a lower daily dose. Or you can take a routine daily dose of 3 to 5 grams. You can get more creatine in your diet by eating animal-based foods like beef and salmon, which provide about 500 milligrams per 4-ounce serving.

BETA-ALANINE: Beta-alanine is an amino acid found in poultry, meat, and fish. Your body uses it to produce carnosine, which serves as an acid buffer and helps improve exercise performance. It also improves muscle fiber firing rates and recovery. This is one that I mostly reserve for my athletes. You really don't need it if you're not competitive, but it may improve your performance if you are.

Carnosine levels are naturally lower in females than males, but females experience greater relative increases in carnosine after beta-alanine supplementation. Studies of female master athletes show performance gains with beta-alanine supplementation, including improvement in lower body exercise performance and in cycling time trial performance. A study of premenopausal soccer players found that beta-alanine supplementation during plyometric training appeared to add further adaptive changes in endurance and repeated sprinting and jumping ability.

For women in the menopausal transition who suffer hot flashes, a dose of beta-alanine, which helps open your blood vessels, before you head out can help ward them off.

Research has shown exercise improvements with consumption of 4 to 6 grams a day. Some people get pins-and-needles sensations at the higher end of that recommended dosage. You can avoid that by taking it in two separate doses over the course of the day.

CAFFEINE: No discussion of ergogenic aids would be complete without a discussion of caffeine. Hands down, caffeine is the most widely used performance-enhancing drug in the world—for athletes and non-athletes alike. It's so popular in endurance sports such as cycling that many teams even have coffee sponsors. There's a good reason it's so popular. It works.

A 2020 meta-analysis and International Society of Sports Nutrition position stand on caffeine in sports concluded that caffeine has a positive effect on exercise performance, including improvement to muscular endurance, movement velocity, muscle strength, sprinting, jumping, throwing, and other aspects of aerobic and anaerobic performance. Caffeine improves cognitive function, especially attention, and it also can sharpen mental and physical performance when you're short on sleep (though caffeine is no substitute for proper shuteye).

Caffeine's main performance benefit is that, as a central nervous system stimulant, it gives you energy so you're ready to go. Caffeine also strengthens your muscle contractions by increasing the calcium content of your muscle, which is just what you need to bang out the last 200 meters in a race or to power through that final set of pull-ups. It also increases your power output and time to exhaustion and lowers your perceived exertion. To put it more simply: caffeine enables you to run, bike, swim, row, or whatever longer and more powerfully, while feeling less tired.

A 2016 analysis found minor sex differences. Women had greater blood pressure increases, but less heart rate changes compared to men. Higher levels of circulating estrogen made women feel the effects of caffeine—such as the jitteriness—more but that didn't change their performance improvements. Research on women shows that caffeine may be more beneficial for longer, sustained endurance exercise than for high-intensity sprints.

There are many forms of caffeine to choose from: coffee, tea, soda, pills, gums, and natural energy shots. Each of these products contains a certain dose of caffeine. For reference, a double espresso delivers about 130 milligrams, 16 ounces of brewed coffee contains about 250 milligrams, and one small Red Bull has about 80 milligrams of caffeine. Caffeine is easily absorbed by the stomach and intestine, so you reach peak blood levels within 45 to 60 minutes after taking it.

How much caffeine you should take depends on your size and tolerance. Generally speaking, the recommended dose ranges from 2 to 6 milligrams of caffeine per kilogram of body weight, or one to two cups of coffee for a 135-pound woman. More is definitely not better; if you're not accustomed to caffeine, start on the low end and see how well you tolerate it. (It can cause jitteriness and GI upset in some people.) As with everything else, if you plan to use caffeine during a big event or competition, be sure you train with it first so you know how your body reacts to it.

For maximum benefits, take your caffeine 45 minutes to an hour before training. If you're an endurance athlete, caffeine is also extremely beneficial during times when you have an accumulation of fatigue. So if you're out for a marathon or a long ride, some caffeinated chews may be just what you need three-quarters of the way through.

COLLAGEN: The jury is still out on collagen. Collagen supplements have been sold (and women have been taking them) for decades in the hope of improving the quality of their skin. Collagen marketers promise that these products can improve skin elasticity, reduce wrinkles, increase blood flow to the skin . . . you know the drill. Though it's true that collagen is one of the primary building blocks of skin, as well as of muscles and connective tissues like ligaments and tendons, it's not clear if collagen supplements actually do much good. Some research suggests that collagen supplements may improve collagen synthesis—that is, they may improve the integrity of your connective tissues—when taken an hour before exercise. But more research is needed to say for sure. If you want to try taking collagen supplements, there's no harm in it. We just can't say for sure if it will really help.

19

PULLING IT ALL TOGETHER

Now it's time to pull it all together. Remember, every woman's menopausal journey is unique. My goal is to arm you with the information you need to make the best decisions for yourself to feel and perform your best. This section will help you take inventory of where you are and map out your menopausal plan of action to get where you want to go!

FIRST, TRACK THE CHANGES

Menopause is a confusing time. Body composition changes can spring up seemingly out of nowhere. Symptoms like irregular periods, mood swings, night sweats, and hot flashes can start five years before your periods stop (and sometimes even earlier!), and new symptoms, especially vaginal dryness and urinary incontinence, can pop up after you're through the transition.

The advice in this book is designed to help you get a handle on it all. To see what is working for you (and maybe what isn't), it's helpful to do some initial self-assessments and then track any changes as you implement exercise, nutrition, and other interventions.

TAKE INVENTORY OF YOUR SYMPTOMS

Let's start with your symptoms. Let's say your sleep has been bad. Is your sleep disrupted every night? Are you having night sweats and racing thoughts? Maybe you're having hot flashes. Do you know how many? How bad are they? When do they usually happen? Have you been feeling "off" in other ways that have you scratching your head, wondering what's wrong with you?

Taking inventory will help you understand what you want to address. It's also helpful to have this inventory handy for doctor's visits or if you pursue menopausal hormone therapy or other pharmaceutical interventions.

Some symptoms to watch for:

- *Irregular menstrual cycles (track cycle timing, length, and bleeding)*
- *Hot flashes (also called hot flushes in some countries)*
- *Night sweats*
- *Weight gain or body composition changes, especially muscle loss and fat gain*
- *Difficulty sleeping*
- *Mood changes—especially depression, anxiety, or anger*
- *Brain fog or forgetfulness*
- *Vaginal dryness (including painful sex) and incontinence*
- *Joint pain*
- *Headaches or migraines*

You can track your symptoms the old-fashioned way with a pen and paper, or you can use one of the many menopause tracking apps that allow you to track dozens of symptoms and their severity.

KEEPING SCORE

The Australian Menopause Society has created a "Symptom Score" chart that can help you keep track of your symptoms and that facilitates a targeted conversation with your health care provider about the treatment options available to you. This chart was designed to be used in conjunction with hormonal therapy, but you can also use it to track how well adaptogens or other interventions are working.

To use the chart, rate the severity of each symptom on a 1 to 3 scale, with 1 for mild, 2 for moderate, 3 for severe; score yourself 0, of course, if you do not have that particular symptom. A score of 15 or higher usually indicates that your symptoms are disruptive enough to require treatment, but this figure is only a guideline. Scores between 20 and 50 are common in symptomatic women. With adequate treatment tailored to the individual, their score can typically be reduced to 10 or under in three to six months. If you're still experiencing a lot of symptoms, you may require another intervention (like a higher dose or another form of MHT).

	Starting Score	Intervention	Score after 6 months
Hot flashes			
Lightheaded feelings			
Headaches			
Irritability			
Depression			
Unloved feelings			
Anxiety			
Mood changes			
Sleeplessness			
Unusual tiredness			
Backache			
Joint pains			
Muscle pains			
New facial hair			
Dry skin			
Crawling feelings under the skin			
Less sexual feelings			
Dry vagina			
Uncomfortable intercourse			
Urinary frequency			
Total:			

The severity of your symptoms is scored as follows:

None = 0

Mild = 1

Moderate = 2

Severe = 3

The symptoms are grouped into four categories: vasomotor, psychological, locomotor, and urogenital. If one group of symptoms do not respond to MHT, look for other causes and specific treatments for that group. Not all of the symptoms listed are necessarily estrogen-deficiency symptoms.

Credit: Australian Menopause Society

BODY COMPOSITION TRACKING

The number-one complaint I hear from menopausal women when they knock on my door is about their body composition. They've lost muscle and gained fat, and they're not very happy about it. Weight is always a sticky subject because there's so much pressure on women, internally and externally, to be a certain size. Some of our sports are power-to-weight-based, so we can be thrown off our game if our power goes down or our weight goes up.

I know that women can become obsessive about weight in ways that are mentally and physically unhealthy. Again, statistics show that roughly 80 percent of women in the United States are unhappy with the way they look. Such feelings are also widespread in athletic populations—maybe even more so.

There's nothing wrong with wanting to improve your body composition—to build strong muscles and lose some unwanted fat—but pouring too much energy into the singular goal of losing weight is not healthy and can often lead to counterproductive behaviors (like fasting!). Also, if you think negatively about your weight every day, day in and day out, you won't feel and perform at your best.

It's important to recognize that *everyone* has body composition changes with age. That is inevitable. We can mitigate some of the sudden shifts that come with menopause, and you absolutely can make body composition changes that will help you feel and perform better. But we cannot promise that your body composition will be the same in your fifties as it was in your thirties.

That's why I recommend focusing your attention on how much muscle you have rather than a number on the scale. I encourage you to track your strength. How much power you can produce on your bike, the weight you can lift in the gym, your pace on the trail, how good you feel—these are the ultimate tests of your progress.

I also recommend working with your somatotype. Everyone has a different body type. Some of us are naturally curvy, while others are naturally muscular or thin. Fighting against your body type can be nothing but an exercise in frustration. Though some people think the concept of somatotypes sounds "new-agey," it, in fact, dates back to ancient Greece and Hippocrates. Dr. William Sheldon introduced the three types that we use today, back in the 1940s. He took it one step further and assigned personality types to each one. The personality types have since been dismissed, but the physical characteristics have held up. Once again, as is often the case, more research needs to be done on women. Nevertheless, sport science research reports that somatotype has a strong influence on sports performance.

Most of us fall into one of three categories:

- *Ectomorph: You tend to be long-limbed and not particularly muscular. You can be thin without necessarily having a lean body composition.*

- *Mesomorph: It is relatively easy for you to build muscle mass. You are medium-boned and proportionally built.*

- *Endomorph: You tend to have a curvier build. You may have larger bone structure, and you store fat relatively easily.*

These are basic types, of course. There are a wide variety of shapes and sizes within these three categories, and you can be a combination of two types rather than just a single type. Common combinations are ecto-endomorphs, who have light upper bodies but greater mass in the hips and thighs (what is commonly called a "pear" shape), and endo-ectomorphs, who have higher mass and fat storage in the torso and midsection and thinner lower bodies (what is commonly called an "apple" shape).

Many factors influence your somatotype, including your genes and ethnicity. Importantly, none of these somatotypes is "superior" or the best one to be. Ectomorphs can train to be strong, and endomorphs are not automatically "overweight" just because they store fat more easily. But understanding your natural build can help guide your goals. If you're an endomorph, you are always going to be more solidly built, and setting a goal to "lose weight" is less useful than setting a goal to optimize your body composition.

Whatever body composition goal you ultimately set, I encourage you to go beyond the bathroom scale. That singular number tells you nothing about your strength and performance. Remember, simply weighing more is not a bad thing. One woman's scale may say 127, but if she is proportionately low in lean muscle, being "lighter" is not "better." As we noted earlier, another woman's scale may read 25 or 30 pounds heavier but she may be out there slaying it in her triathlons or in the gym because she is literally being powered by strong muscle mass.

Likewise, body mass index (BMI), which became a popular health metric in the 1990s, has been largely debunked as a useful calculation for health and performance. One large meta-analysis even concluded that people with BMIs that fell into the "overweight" category (BMI of 25 to 29.9) had the lowest risk of dying early from any cause. And even people with BMIs that fell into the "obese" range (BMI of 30 to 34.9) were not at any higher risk of early death. BMI, which is calculated by dividing your weight in kilograms by your height in meters squared, is particularly problematic for active people, who tend to have a higher proportion of muscle tissue, which is denser than fat. Muscle mass can make a woman's weight relatively high for her size.

If you are motivated by data and want some numbers by which to measure progress, go with body composition, which is a measure of fat mass to lean tissue. A healthy range is anywhere from around 19 to 32 percent body fat, depending on your age. For athletic purposes, the ranges skew a bit lower, as the American College of Sports Medicine's chart indicates. Menopausal women will naturally have more fat (as you can also see in the chart). That is normal and healthy.

Fitness category	Age (years)				
	20-29	30-39	40-49	50-59	60+
Essential fat	10-13	10-13	10-13	10-13	10-13
Excellent	14.5-17	15.5-17.9	18.5-21.2	21.6-24.9	21.1-25
Good	17.1-20.5	18.5-21.2	21.3-24.8	25-28.4	25.1-29.2
Average	20.6-23.6	21.6-24.8	24.9-28	28.5-31.5	29.3-32.4
Below average	23.7-27.6	24.9-29.2	28.1-32	31.6-35.5	32.5-36.5
Poor	>27.7	>29.3	>32.1	>35.6	>36.6

SCHEDULING YOUR TRAINING

One of the hardest parts of training isn't knowing what to do—it's knowing when to do it. You know you need to lift heavy sh*t, and you know you need SIT training. You want truly hard days and truly easy days with less time spent in the gray area—that place where you're working just hard enough to get worn down, but not hard enough to gain the training stimulus you need to see progress. And of course, if you're an endurance athlete, you want to make room for those two-hour runs and three-hour rides and all the stuff you love.

How to put it all together? This depends somewhat on your preferences, your work schedule, and how you respond to training. Some women do best with easy days breaking up the hard days. Others prefer stacking hard days back to back and then scheduling a longer stretch of moderate and easy days. Ultimately, you'll need to experiment a bit to find what works best for you. Here are two schemes that I recommend:

Alternate Day Scheme:

Monday	Tuesday	Wednesday	Thursday	Friday	Saturday	Sunday
Rest day	SIT intervals LHS session (total body)	Easy training day: yoga, functional mobility, cardio, etc.	SIT intervals LHS session (total body)	Rest day or easy active recovery	Endurance day	Endurance day

Hard Block Scheme:

Monday	Tuesday	Wednesday	Thursday	Friday	Saturday	Sunday
SIT intervals LHS session (lower body)	SIT intervals LHS session (upper body/core)	Easy training day: yoga, functional mobility, cardio, etc.	Moderate cardio or body weight circuit training	Rest day or easy active recovery	Longer endurance or circuit training	Rest day or easy active recovery

PLANNING YOUR NUTRITION

As we discussed, most active women do not eat enough. When you put your body in a state of low energy availability, you hang on to fat and lose muscle—the exact opposite of what you want. Active women need at least 2,000 calories a day, not including the snacks they need during long rides or runs. Those calories should come from mostly carbs and protein in about equal amounts on easy days and from slightly more carbs, along with a healthy dose of fat (which you generally get naturally), on moderate to hard training days.

It's good to have a general idea of how much of each macronutrient you're getting. And remember, timing is important. Too many women eat little to nothing early in the day and then devour all their calories at dinner and later. This is counterproductive, especially if you're menopausal, because you need more protein to make and maintain muscle and your body can only process so much at one sitting. You also need carbs to fuel your workouts, which, if you're like most athletes, generally happen earlier in the day. Eating a big meal later in the day also can fill your digestive system too close to bed, disrupting your sleep. Ideally, you want to avoid eating within two hours of bedtime.

Here are some carbohydrate/protein guidelines to get you started:

CARBOHYDRATES

Your stored glycogen (carbs) is very limited. Did you know:

- When your muscle glycogen stores are used up, you become exhausted.
- Muscle glycogen depletion occurs after two to three hours of continuous low-intensity training, but within 15 to 30 minutes of high-intensity training.
- When liver glycogen is depleted, your body cannot keep your blood glucose levels normal. This is when you hit the wall and cannot continue.
- With low blood glucose levels, your body has to rely on fat for fuel; however, this is a very slow process, and it will limit your activity.
- Signs and symptoms of low blood glucose include light-headedness, lack of coordination, weakness, inability to concentrate, blurry vision, and a spacey feeling.

HOW MANY CARBOHYDRATES DO YOU NEED IN A DAY?

- Menopausal athletes should prioritize carbohydrate intake around (pre, during, post) training, especially high intensity sessions. How much you need depends on your training for the day.
- For moderate- to high-intensity training lasting 60 to 120 minutes, you need 3 to 3.5 grams of carbohydrates per kilogram. For a light or active recovery day, aim for 2.5 grams per kilogram. For short intense days (like CrossFit training), aim for 2.5 to 3 grams of carbs per kilogram.
- For endurance training involving two to five hours of intense training per day (distance running, cycling, swimming), you need 5 to 6 grams

of carbs per kilogram. Again, consume in and around your training sessions.

- For extreme intense training of five hours or more per day (Ironman or multisport events), you need 6 to 8 grams of carbs per kilogram.

My activity per day is: _____

My weight in kilograms (1 kilogram = 2.2 pounds) is: _____

My carbohydrate need (weight in kilograms) x (grams of carb for activity level) is:

_____

PROTEIN

For general muscle growth, repair, and strength adaptations, protein is the key to success! Did you know that:

- In activities lasting two hours or more, amino acids (the building blocks of protein) can give you up to 5 to 10 percent of the fuel necessary to keep going.

- Hydration is key with any endurance activity, and the amino acids of protein are an effective rehydration mechanism.

- Endurance and strength athletes need upward of two grams of protein per kilogram a day for optimal muscle repair, growth, recovery, and fat mobilization.

- If you don't eat any protein, your body will not use carbohydrates for refueling muscle and liver glycogen, as it is supposed to; instead, the carbs you eat will assist in repairing your muscles.

- Protein is also necessary to facilitate fat loss, as it keeps the muscles repairing and rebuilding, a process that allows carbohydrates to refuel the muscles and liver—thus allowing fat stores to stay empty.

HOW MUCH PROTEIN DO YOU NEED IN A DAY?

- For strength and power phases of training, you need 2.0 to 2.2 grams of protein per kilogram.

- For endurance phases of training, you need 1.8 to 2.0 grams of protein per kilogram.

- For optimal recovery, try to take in 30 to 40 grams of protein within the first half-hour after an event or training session.

- For a nontraining day, aim for to 1.8 grams per kilogram.

- To stimulate maximal muscle protein synthesis (a.k.a. make the most muscle), aim for a per-meal dose of 0.5 to 0.6 grams of quality protein per kilogram.

My phase of training is: _____

My weight (1 kilogram = 2.2 pounds) is: _____

My protein need (weight in kilograms x grams of protein for phase of training) is:

_____

HOW TO DO IT

It's very hard to make sweeping changes all at once. So take this month to implement these nutrition strategies in a manageable, stepwise fashion.

WEEK 1: PRIORITIZE PROTEIN

Aim for 30 to 35 grams of protein at each meal and 15 to 20 grams at your snacks. Time it so that you get your biggest protein hit—about 30 to 40 grams—after your daily workout, when your body is primed to use it. Lean meat packs a lot of protein, but you also can get your protein from plant foods like Greek yogurt, nut butters, and edamame and soy foods. Take this week to track your protein timing and intake.

Monday	Tuesday	Wednesday	Thursday	Friday	Saturday	Sunday
Breakfast ____ grams	Breakfast ____ grams	Breakfast ____ grams	Breakfast ____ grams	Breakfast ____ grams	Breakfast ____ grams	Breakfast ____ grams
Snack ____ grams	Snack ____ grams	Snack ____ grams	Snack ____ grams	Snack ____ grams	Snack ____ grams	Snack ____ grams
Lunch ____ grams	Lunch ____ grams	Lunch ____ grams	Lunch ____ grams	Lunch ____ grams	Lunch ____ grams	Lunch ____ grams
Snack ____ grams	Snack ____ grams	Snack ____ grams	Snack ____ grams	Snack ____ grams	Snack ____ grams	Snack ____ grams
Dinner ____ grams	Dinner ____ grams	Dinner ____ grams	Dinner ____ grams	Dinner ____ grams	Dinner ____ grams	Dinner ____ grams

WEEK 2: CONCENTRATE ON QUALITY CARBS

It's important to focus on the quality and timing of your carbohydrates. Eat the bulk of your carbs in the form of fruits and vegetables (and yes, root veggies like sweet potatoes count!). Take this week to track your carbohydrate types and timing. Focus on replacing your usual standbys like pasta and bagels with more nutrient- and fiber-dense, carbohydrate-rich foods.

	Monday	Tuesday	Wednesday	Thursday	Friday	Saturday	Sunday
Carbs eaten today							
Type _____ Time _____							
Type _____ Time _____							
Type _____ Time _____							
Type _____ Time _____							
Type _____ Time _____							

WEEK 3: TAKE A LOOK AT YOUR TIMING

Your goals this week are to move your eating up in the day; to spread your nutrition more evenly throughout the day so that you have the energy you need for your workouts and proper recovery afterward; and to leave two hours before your last meal and bedtime.

Monday	Tuesday	Wednesday	Thursday	Friday	Saturday	Sunday
Breakfast time	Breakfast time	Breakfast time	Breakfast time	Breakfast time	Breakfast time	Breakfast time
Snack time	Snack time	Snack time	Snack time	Snack time	Snack time	Snack time
Lunch time	Lunch time	Lunch time	Lunch time	Lunch time	Lunch time	Lunch time
Snack time	Snack time	Snack time	Snack time	Snack time	Snack time	Snack time
Dinner time	Dinner time	Dinner time	Dinner time	Dinner time	Dinner time	Dinner time
Bedtime How was your sleep?	Bedtime How was your sleep?	Bedtime How was your sleep?	Bedtime How was your sleep?	Bedtime How was your sleep?	Bedtime How was your sleep?	Bedtime How was your sleep?
Exercise type/time How did you feel?	Exercise type/time How did you feel?	Exercise type/time How did you feel?	Exercise type/time How did you feel?	Exercise type/time How did you feel?	Exercise type/time How did you feel?	Exercise type/time How did you feel?

WEEK 4: ASSESS YOUR PROGRESS AND PULL IT ALL TOGETHER

This week give yourself a pat on the back for applying yourself to these healthy changes. Go back and assess what worked and what didn't, then make adjustments as you take this week to try to pull it all together. Well done!

BIBLIOGRAPHY

Below are the primary sources used in each chapter. More sources can be found online at drstacysims.com/nextlevel.

2: THE SCIENCE OF THE MENOPAUSE TRANSITION

Baltasar, Lucía Vázquez, and Ana Belén Flórez. "Equol: A Bacterial Metabolite from the Daidzein Isoflavone and Its Presumed Beneficial Health Effects." *Nutrients* 11, no. 9 (2019): 2231. www.ncbi.nlm.nih.gov/pmc/articles/PMC6770660.

Finkelstein, Joel S., Hang Lee, Arun Karlamangla, Robert M. Neer, Patrick M. Sluss, Sherri-Ann M. Burnett-Bowie, Karin Darakananda, et al. "Antimullerian Hormone and Impending Menopause in Late Reproductive Age: The Study of Women's Health Across the Nation." *Journal of Clinical Endocrinology & Metabolism* 105, no. 4 (2020): e1862–e1871. https://academic.oup.com/jcem/article-abstract/105/4/e1862/5709648?redirectedFrom=fulltext.

Gaya, Pilar, Margarita Medina, Abel Sánchez-Jiménez, and José María Landete. "Phytoestrogen Metabolism by Adult Human Gut Microbiota." *Molecules* 21, no. 8 (2016): 1034. www.mdpi.com/1420-3049/21/8/1034.

Green, R., A. J. Polotsky, R. P. Wildman, A. P. McGinn, J. Lin, C. Derby, J. Johnston, et al. "Menopausal Symptoms Within a Hispanic Cohort: SWAN, the Study of Women's Health Across the Nation." *Women's Health* 5, no. 2 (2009): 127–33. www.ncbi.nlm.nih.gov/pmc/articles/PMC3270699.

Kroenke, Candyce H., Bette J. Caan, Marcia L. Stefanick, Garnet Anderson, Robert Brzyski, Karen C. Johnson, Erin LeBlanc, et al. "Effects of a Dietary Intervention and Weight Change on Vasomotor Symptoms in the Women's Health Initiative." *Menopause* 19, no. 9 (2013): 980–88. www.ncbi.nlm.nih.gov/pmc/articles/PMC3428489.

Rafii, Fatemeh. "The Role of Colonic Bacteria in the Metabolism of the Natural Isoflavone Daidzin to Equol." *Metabolites* 5, no. 1 (2015): 56–73. www.ncbi.nlm.nih.gov/pmc/articles/PMC4381290.

Reed, Susan D., Johanna W. Lampe, Conghui Qu, Wade K. Copeland, Gabrielle Gundersen, Sharon Fuller, and Katherine M. Newton. "Premenopausal Vasomotor Symptoms in an Ethnically Diverse Population." *Menopause* 21, no. 2 (2014): 153–58. Baltasar Mayo, https://pubmed.ncbi.nlm.nih.gov/23760434.

Sternfeld, Barbara, Katherine A. Guthrie, Kristine E. Ensrud, Andrea Z. LaCroix, Joseph C. Larson, Andrea L. Dunn, Garnet L. Anderson, et al. "Efficacy of Exercise for Menopausal Symptoms: A Randomized Controlled Trial." *Menopause* 21, no. 4 (2014): 330–38. www.ncbi.nlm.nih.gov/pmc/articles/PMC3858421.

3: HORMONES AND SYMPTOMS EXPLAINED

Bereshchenko, Oxana, Stefano Bruscoli, and Carlo Riccardi. "Glucocorticoids, Sex Hormones, and Immunity." *Frontiers in Immunology* 9 (June 2018): 1332. www.ncbi.nlm.nih.gov/pmc/articles/PMC6006719.

Campello, Raquel S., Luciana A. Fátima, João Nilton Barreto-Andrade, Thais F. Lucas, Rosana C. Mori, Catarina S. Porto, and Ubiratan F. Machado. "Estradiol-Induced Regulation of GLUT4 in 3T3-L1 Cells: Involvement of ESR1 and AKT Activation." *Journal of Molecular Endocrinology* 59, no. 3 (2017): 257–68. https://pubmed.ncbi.nlm.nih.gov/28729437.

Hall, Olivia J., and Sabra L. Klein. "Progesterone-Based Compounds Affect Immune Responses and Susceptibility to Infections at Diverse Mucosal Sites." *Mucosal Immunology* 10, no. 5 (2017): 1097–1107. www.nature.com/articles/mi201735.pdf.

Hudon Thibeault, Andrée-Anne, J. Thomas Sanderson, and Cathy Vaillancourt. "Serotonin-Estrogen Interactions: What Can We Learn from Pregnancy?" *Biochimie* 161 (June 2019): 88–108. www.sciencedirect.com/science/article/abs/pii/S0300908419301002.

Schertzinger, Meredith, Kate Wesson-Sides, Luke Parkitny, and Jarred Younger. "Daily Fluctuations of Progesterone and Testosterone Are Associated with Fibromyalgia Pain Severity." *Journal of Pain* 19, no. 4 (2018): 410–17. www.ncbi.nlm.nih.gov/pmc/articles/PMC6046191.

Shi, Jie, Zhen Yang, Yixin Niu, Weiwei Zhang, Ning Lin, Xiaoyong Li, Hongmei Zhang, et al. "Large Thigh Circumference Is Associated with Lower Blood Pressure in Overweight and Obese Individuals: A Community-Based Study." *Endocrine Connections* 9, no. 4 (2020):271–78. https://pubmed.ncbi.nlm.nih.gov/32247281.

Srikanthan, Preethi, Tamara B. Horwich, Marcella Calfon Press, Jeff Gornbein, and Karol E. Watson. "Sex Differences in the Association of Body Composition and Cardiovascular Mortality." *Journal of the American Heart Association* 10, no. 5 (2021). www.ahajournals.org/doi/10.1161/JAHA.120.017511.

Vincent, Katy, Charlotte J. Stagg, Catherine E. Warnaby, Jane Moore, Stephen Kennedy, and Irene Tracey. "'Luteal Analgesia': Progesterone Dissociates Pain Intensity and Unpleasantness by Influencing Emotion Regulation Networks." *Frontiers in Endocrinology* 9 (July 2018): 413. www.ncbi.nlm.nih.gov/pmc/articles/PMC6064935.

4: MENOPAUSAL HORMONE THERAPY, ADAPTOGENS, AND OTHER INVENTIONS

Auddy, Biswajit, Jayaram Hazra, Achintya Mitra, Bruce Abedon, and Shibnath Ghosal. "A Standardized Withania Somnifera Extract Significantly Reduces Stress-Related Parameters in Chronically Stressed Humans: A Double-Blind, Randomized, Placebo-Controlled Study." *JANA* 11, no. 1 (2008): 50–56. https://blog.priceplow.com/wp-content/uploads/2014/08/withania_review.pdf.

Chester, Rebecca C., Juliana M. Kling, and Joann E. Manson. "What the Women's Health Initiative Has Taught Us About Menopausal Hormone Therapy." *Clinical Cardiology* 41, no. 2 (2018): 247–52. www.ncbi.nlm.nih.gov/pmc/articles/PMC6490107.

Dording, Christina M., Pamela J. Schettler, Elizabeth D. Dalton, Susannah R. Parkin, Rosemary S. W. Walker, Kara B. Fehling, Maurizio Fava, et al. "A Double-Blind Placebo-Controlled Trial of Maca Root as Treatment for Antidepressant-Induced Sexual Dysfunction in Women." *Evidence-Based Complementary and Alternative Medicine* (April 14, 2015). www.ncbi.nlm.nih.gov/pmc/articles/PMC4411442.

Gerbarg, Patricia L., and Richard P. Brown. "Pause Menopause with Rhodiola Rosea, a Natural Selective Estrogen Receptor Modulator." *Phytomedicine: International Journal of Phytotherapy and Phytopharmacology* 23, no. 7 (2016): 763–69. https://pubmed.ncbi.nlm.nih.gov/26776957.

Ishaque, Sana, Larissa Shamseer, Cecilia Bukutu, and Sunita Vohra. "Rhodiola rosea for Physical and Mental Fatigue: A Systematic Review." *BMC Complementary and Alternative Medicine* 12 (May 2012): 70. www.ncbi.nlm.nih.gov/pmc/articles/PMC3541197.

Jamshidi, Negar, and Marc M. Cohen. "The Clinical Efficacy and Safety of Tulsi in Humans: A Systematic Review of the Literature." *Evidence-Based Complementary and Alternative Medicine* (March 16, 2017). www.hindawi.com/journals/ecam/2017/9217567.

Kim, Mi Hye, Hyoun-Su Lee, Seong Bin Hong, and Woong Mo Yang. "Schizandra chinensis Exhibits Phytoestrogenic Effects by Regulating the Activation of Estrogen Receptor-A and -B." *Chinese Journal of Integrative Medicine* (July 31, 2017). https://pubmed.ncbi.nlm.nih.gov/28762131.

Lopresti, Adrian L. Stephen J. Smith, Hakeemudin Malvi, and Rahul Kodgule. "An Investigation into the Stress-Relieving and Pharmacological Actions of an Ashwagandha (Withania Somnifera) Extract." *Medicine* (Baltimore) 98, no. 37 (2019). https://www.ncbi.nlm.nih.gov/pmc/articles/PMC6750292.

Mehta, Jaya, Juliana M. Kling, and JoAnn E. Manson. "Risks, Benefits, and Treatment Modalities of Menopausal Hormone Therapy: Current Concepts." *Frontiers in Endocrinology* 12 (March 26, 2021). https://doi.org/10.3389/fendo.2021.564781.

Meissner, H. O., W. Kapczynski, A. Mscisz, and J. Lutomski. "Use of Gelatinized Maca (Lepidium Peruvianum) in Early Postmenopausal Women." *International Journal of Biomedical Science* 1, no. 1 (2005): 33–45. www.ncbi.nlm.nih.gov/pmc/articles/PMC3614576.

Million Women Study Collaborators. "Breast Cancer and Hormone-Replacement Therapy in the Million Women Study." *Lancet* 362, no. 9382 (2003). www.thelancet.com/journals/lancet/article/PIIS0140-6736(03)14065-2/ fulltext.

Modi, Mansi B., Shilpa B. Donga, and Laxmipriya Dei. "Clinical Evaluation of Ashokarishta, Ashwagandha Churna and Praval Pishti in the Management of Menopausal Syndrome." *Ayu* 33, no. 4 (2012): 511–16. www.ncbi.nlm .nih.gov/pmc/articles/PMC3665193.

Palacios, Santiago, John C. Stevenson, Katrin Schaudig, Monika Lukasiewicz, and Alessandra Graziottin. "Hormone Therapy for First-Line Management of Menopausal Symptoms: Practical Recommendations." *Women's Health* (London) 15 (August 2019). www.ncbi.nlm.nih.gov/pmc/articles/PMC6683316.

Park, J. Y., and K. H. Kim. "A Randomized, Double-Blind, Placebo-Controlled Trial of Schisandra chinensis for Menopausal Symptoms." *Climacteric: The Journal of the International Menopause Society* 19, no. 6 (2016): 574– 80. https://pubmed.ncbi.nlm.nih.gov/27763802.

Raut, Ashwinikumar A., Nirmala N. Rege, Firoz M. Tadvi, Punita V. Solanki, Kirti R. Kene, Sudatta G. Shirolkar, Shefali N. Pandey, et al. "Exploratory Study to Evaluate Tolerability, Safety, and Activity of Ashwagandha (Withania Somnifera) in Healthy Volunteers." *Journal of Ayurveda and Integrative Medicine* 3, no. 3 (2012): 111– 14. www.ncbi.nlm.nih.gov/pmc/articles/PMC3487234.

Salve, Jaysing, Sucheta Pate, Khokan Debnath, and Deepak Langade. "Adaptogenic and Anxiolytic Effects of Ashwagandha Root Extract in Healthy Adults: A Double-Blind, Randomized, Placebo-Controlled Clinical Study." *Cureus* 11, no. 12 (2019). www.ncbi.nlm.nih.gov/pmc/articles/PMC6979308.

Santoro, Nanette, Arthur Waldbaum, Samuel Lederman, Robin Kroll, Graeme L. Fraser, Christopher Lademacher, Laurence Skillern, et al. "Effect of the Neurokinin 3 Receptor Antagonist Fezolinetant on Patient-Reported Outcomes in Postmenopausal Women with Vasomotor Symptoms: Results of a Randomized, Placebo-Controlled, Double-Blind, Dose-Ranging Study (VESTA)." *Menopause* 27, no. 12 (2020): 1350–56. www.ncbi.nlm .nih.gov/pmc/articles/PMC7709922.

Szopa, Agnieszka, Radosław Ekiert, and Halina Ekiert. "Current Knowledge of Schisandra chinensis (Turcz.) Baill. (Chinese Magnolia Vine) As a Medicinal Plant Species: A Review on the Bioactive Components, Pharmacological Properties, Analytical and Biotechnological Studies. *Phytochemistry Reviews* 16 (April 2017): 195–218. https://link.springer.com/article/10.1007/s11101-016-9470-4.

Vinogradova, Yana, Carol Coupland, and Julia Hippisley-Cox. "Use of Hormone Replacement Therapy and Risk of Breast Cancer: Nested Case-Control Studies Using the Qresearch and CPRD Databases." *BMJ* (October 28, 2020): 371. www.bmj.com/content/371/bmj.m3873.

5: KICK UP YOUR CARDIO

Boutcher, Yati N., Stephen H. Boutcher, Hye Y. Yoo, and Jarrod D. Meerkin. "The Effect of Sprint Interval Training on Body Composition of Postmenopausal Women." *Medicine and Science in Sports and Exercise* 51, no. 7 (2019):1413–19. https://europepmc.org/article/med/31210647.

Buckinx, Fanny, and Mylène Aubertin-Leheudre. "Menopause and High-Intensity Interval Training: Effects on Body Composition and Physical Performance." *Menopause* 26, no. 11 (2019): 1232–33. https://journals.lww.com /menopausejournal/Citation/2019/11000/Menopause_and_high_intensity_interval_training_.2.aspx.

Dupuit, Marine, Florie Maillard, Bruno Pereira, Marcelo Luis Marquezi, Antonio Herbert Lancha Jr., and Nathalie Boisseau. "Effect of High Intensity Interval Training on Body Composition in Women Before and After Menopause: A Meta-Analysis." *Experimental Physiology* 105, no. 9 (2020): 1470–90. https://physoc.onlinelibrary .wiley.com/doi/10.1113/EP088654.

Gillen, Jenna B., Brian J. Martin, Martin J. MacInnis, Lauren E. Skelly, Mark A. Tarnopolsky, and Martin J. Gibala. "Twelve Weeks of Sprint Interval Training Improves Indices of Cardiometabolic Health Similar to Traditional Endurance Training Despite a Five-Fold Lower Exercise Volume and Time Commitment." *PLoS One* 11, no. 4 (2016). https://journals.plos.org/plosone/article?id=10.1371/journal.pone.0154075.

Klonizakis, Markos, James Moss, Stephen Gilbert, David Broom, Jeff Foster, and Garry A. Tew. "Low-Volume High-Intensity Interval Training Rapidly Improves Cardiopulmonary Function in Postmenopausal Women." *Menopause* 21, no. 10 (2014): 1099–1105. https://pubmed.ncbi.nlm.nih.gov/24552980.

Maillard, F., S. Rousset, B. Pereira, A. Traore, P. de Pradel Del Amaze, Y. Boirie, M. Duclos, et al. "High-Intensity Interval Training Reduces Abdominal Fat Mass in Postmenopausal Women with Type 2 Diabetes." *Diabetes & Metabolism* 42, no. 6 (2016): 433–41. https://pubmed.ncbi.nlm.nih.gov/27567125.

Sylwester, Kujach, Olek Robert Antoni, Byun Kyeongho, Suwabe Kazuya, Sitek Emilia J., Ziemann Ewa, Laskowski Radosław, and Soya Hideaki. "Acute Sprint Interval Exercise Increases Both Cognitive Functions and Peripheral Neurotrophic Factors in Humans: The Possible Involvement of Lactate." *Frontiers in Neuroscience* 12 (January 23, 2020). www.frontiersin.org/articles/10.3389/fnins.2019.01455/full.

6: NOW'S THE TIME TO LIFT HEAVY SH*T!

Abildgaard, J., A. T. Pedersen, C. J. Green, N. M. Harder-Lauridsen, T. P. Solomon, C. Thomsen, A. Juul, M. Pedersen, et al. "Menopause Is Associated with Decreased Whole Body Fat Oxidation During Exercise." *American Journal of Physiology-Endocrinology and Metabolism* 304, no. 11 (2013): E1227–E1236. https://journals.physiology.org/doi/full/10.1152/ajpendo.00492.2012.

Collins, Brittany C., Robert W. Arpke, Alexie A. Larson, Cory W. Baumann, Ning Xie, Christine A. Cabelka, Nardina L. Nash, et al. "Estrogen Regulates the Satellite Cell Compartment in Females." *Cell Reports* 28, no. 2 (2019): 368–81. www.ncbi.nlm.nih.gov/pmc/articles/PMC6655560.

Li, Fei, George P. Nassis, Yue Shi, Guangqiang Han, Xiaohui Zhang, Binghong Gao, and Haiyong Ding. "Concurrent Complex and Endurance Training for Recreational Marathon Runners: Effects on Neuromuscular and Running Performance." *European Journal of Sport Science* 21, no. 9 (2021): 1243–53. https://pubmed.ncbi.nlm.nih.gov/32981468.

Sunde, Arnstein, Oyvind Støren, Marius Bjerkaas, Morten H. Larsen, Jan Hoff, and Jan Helgerud. "Maximal Strength Training Improves Cycling Economy in Competitive Cyclists." *Journal of Strength and Conditioning Research* 24, no. 8 (2010): 2157–65. https://pubmed.ncbi.nlm.nih.gov/19855311.

7: GET A JUMP ON MENOPAUSAL STRENGTH LOSSES

Hinton, Pamela S., Peggy Nigh, and John Thyfault. "Effectiveness of Resistance Training or Jumping-Exercise to Increase Bone Mineral Density in Men with Low Bone Mass: A 12-Month Randomized, Clinical Trial." *Bone* 79 (October 2015): 203–12. www.ncbi.nlm.nih.gov/pmc/articles/PMC4503233.

Smale, K. B., L. H. Hansen, J. K. Kristensen, M. K. Zebis, C. Andersen, D. L. Benoit, E. W. Helge, and T. Alkjaer. "Loading Intensity of Jumping Exercises in Post-Menopausal Women: Implications for Osteogenic Training." *Translational Sports Medicine* 1, no. 1 (2018): 30–36. https://onlinelibrary.wiley.com/doi/abs/10.1002/tsm2.5.

Tucker, Larry A., J. Eric Strong, James D. LeCheminant, and Bruce W. Bailey. "Effect of Two Jumping Programs on Hip Bone Mineral Density in Premenopausal Women: A Randomized Controlled Trial." *American Journal of Health Promotion* 29, no. 3 (2015): 158–64. https://journals.sagepub.com/doi/10.4278/ajhp.130430-QUAN-200.

Vetrovsky, Tomas, Michal Steffl, Petr Stastny, and James J. Tufano. "The Efficacy and Safety of Lower-Limb Plyometric Training in Older Adults: A Systematic Review." *Sports Medicine* 49, 113–31. https://link.springer.com/article/10.1007/s40279-018-1018-x.

8: GUT HEALTH FOR ATHLETIC GLORY

Alang, Neha, and Colleen R. Kelly. "Weight Gain After Fecal Microbiota Transplantation." *Open Forum Infectious Diseases* 2, no. 1 (2015). https://academic.oup.com/ofid/article/2/1/ofv004/1461242.

Asnicar, Francesco, Sarah E. Berry, Ana M. Valdes, Long H. Nguyen, Gianmarco Piccinno, David A. Drew, Emily Leeming, et al. "Microbiome Connections with Host Metabolism and Habitual Diet from 1,098 Deeply Phenotyped Individuals." *Nature Medicine* 27 (January 2021): 321–32. http://dx.doi.org/10.1038/s41591-020-01183-8.

Barton, Wiley, Nicholas C. Penney, Owen Cronin, Isabel Garcia-Perez, Michael G. Molloy, Elaine Holmes, Fergus Shanahan, Paul D. Cotter, Orla O'Sullivan. "The Microbiome of Professional Athletes Differs from That of

More Sedentary Subjects in Composition and Particularly at the Functional Metabolic Level." *Gut* 67 (2018): 625–33. https://gut.bmj.com/content/67/4/625.

Crovesy, Louise, Daniele Masterson, and Eliane Lopes Rosado. "Profile of the Gut Microbiota of Adults with Obesity: A Systematic Review." *European Journal of Clinical Nutrition* 74 (March 2020): 1251–62. www.nature .com/articles/s41430-020-0607-6.

Diener, Christian, Shizhen Qin, Yong Zhou, Sushmita Patwardhan, Li Tang, Jennifer C. Lovejoy, Andrew T. Magis, Nathan D. Price, Leroy Hood, and Sean M. Gibbons. "Signature Associated with Variable Weight Loss Responses Following a Healthy Lifestyle Intervention in Humans." *mSystems* 6, no. 5 (2021). https://journals .asm.org/doi/10.1128/mSystems.00964-21.

Li, Yuanyuan, Yanli Hao, Fang Fan, and Bin Zhang. "The Role of Microbiome in Insomnia, Circadian Disturbance and Depression." *Frontiers in Psychiatry* 9 (December 2018): 669. www.ncbi.nlm.nih.gov/pmc/articles /PMC6290721.

Mach, Núria, and Dolor Fuster-Botella. "Endurance Exercise and Gut Microbiota: A Review." *Journal of Sport and Health Science* 62, no. 2 (2017): 179–197. www.ncbi.nlm.nih.gov/pmc/articles/PMC6188999.

Maqsood, Raeesah, and Trevor W. Stone. "The Gut-Brain Axis, BDNF, NMDA and CNS Disorders." *Neurochemical Research* 41, no. 11 (2016): 2819–35. https://pubmed.ncbi.nlm.nih.gov/27553784/#:~:text=Gutmicrobiotacanmod ulateBDNF,(SCFAs)inthebrain.

Mesnage, Robin, Franziska Grundler, Andreas Schwiertz, Yvon Le Maho, and Françoise Wilhelmi de Toledo. "Changes in Human Gut Microbiota Composition Are Linked to the Energy Metabolic Switch During 10 D of Buchinger Fasting." *Journal of Nutritional Science* 8 (November 2019). www.ncbi.nlm.nih.gov/pmc/articles /PMC6861737.

Rinninella, Emanuele, Pauline Raoul, Marco Cintoni, Francesco Franceschi, Giacinto Abele Donato Miggiano, Antonio Gasbarrini, and Maria Cristina Mele. "What Is the Healthy Gut Microbiota Composition? A Changing Ecosystem across Age, Environment, Diet, and Diseases." *Microorganisms* 71, no. 1 (2019): 14. www.ncbi.nlm.nih .gov/pmc/articles/PMC6351938.

Scheiman, Jonathan, Jacob M. Luber, Theodore A. Chavkin, Tara MacDonald, Angela Tung, Loc-Duyen Pham, Marsha C. Wibowo, et al. "Meta-omics Analysis of Elite Athletes Identifies a Performance-Enhancing Microbe That Functions Via Lactate Metabolism." *Nature Medicine* 25 (June 2019): 1104–9. www.nature.com/articles /s41591-019-0485-4.

Suez, Jotham, Tal Korem, David Zeevi, Gili Zilberman-Schapira, Christoph A. Thaiss, Ori Maza, David Israeli, et al. "Artificial Sweeteners Induce Glucose Intolerance by Altering the Gut Microbiota." *Nature* 514 (September 2014): 181–86. www.nature.com/articles/nature13793.

Verdam, Froukje J., Susana Fuentes, Charlotte de Jonge, Erwin G. Zoetendal, Runi Erbil, Jan Willem Greve, Wim A. Buurman, Willem M. de Vos, and Sander S. Rensen. "Human Intestinal Microbiota Composition Is Associated with Local and Systemic Inflammation in Obesity." *Obesity* 21, no. 12 (2013): E607– E615. https:// onlinelibrary.wiley.com/doi/pdf/10.1002/oby.20466.

9: EAT ENOUGH!

Aksungar, Fehime Benli, Aynur Eren, Sengul Ure, Onder Teskin, and Gursel Ates. "Effects of Intermittent Fasting on Serum Lipid Levels, Coagulation Status and Plasma Homocysteine Levels." *Annals of Nutrition & Metabolism* 49, no. 2 (2005): 77–82. https://pubmed.ncbi.nlm.nih.gov/15802901.

Andreotti, Diana Zukas, Silva Josiane do Nascimento, Matumoto Amanda Midori, Orellana Ana Maria, de Mello Paloma Segura, and Kawamoto Elisa Mitiko. "Effects of Physical Exercise on Autophagy and Apoptosis in Aged Brain: Human and Animal Studies." *Frontiers in Nutrition* 7 (July 2020). www.frontiersin.org/articles/10.3389 /fnut.2020.00094/full#h9.

Blick Hoyenga, Katharine, and Kermit T. Hoyenga. "Gender and Energy Balance: Sex Differences in Adaptations for Feast and Famine." *Physiology & Behavior* 28, no. 3 (1982): 545–63. https://doi.org/10.1016/0031 -9384(82)90153-6.

Chella Krishnan, Karthickeyan, Margarete Mehrabian, and Aldons J. Lusis. "Sex Differences in Metabolism and Cardiometabolic Disorders." *Current Opinion in Lipidology* 29, no. 5 (2018): 404–10. www.ncbi.nlm.nih.gov/pmc /articles/PMC6382080.

Cochran, Jesse, Paul V. Taufalele, Kevin D. Lin, Yuan Zhang, and E. Dale Abel. "Sex Differences in the Response of C57BL/6 Mice to Ketogenic Diets." *Diabetes* 67 (suppl. 1) (July 2018). https://diabetes.diabetesjournals.org /content/67/Supplement_1/1884-P.

De Bond, Julie-Ann P., and Jeremy T Smith. "Kisspeptin and energy balance in reproduction." *Reproduction* 147, no. 3 (2014): R53–R63. https://rep.bioscientifica.com/view/journals/rep/147/3/R53.xml.

Dipla, Konstantina, Robert R. Kraemer, Naama W. Constantini, and Anthony C. Hackney. "Relative Energy Deficiency in Sports (RED-S): Elucidation of Endocrine Changes Affecting the Health of Males and Females." *Hormones* (Athens, Greece) 20, no. 1 (2021): 35–47. https://pubmed.ncbi.nlm.nih.gov/32557402.

Durkalec-Michalski, Krzysztof, Paulina M. Nowaczyk, and Katarzyna Siedzik. "Effect of a Four-Week Ketogenic Diet on Exercise Metabolism in CrossFit-Trained Athletes." *Journal of the International Society of Sports Nutrition* 16 (April 2019). https://jissn.biomedcentral.com/articles/10.1186/s12970-019-0284-9.

Fahrenholtz, I. L., A. Sjödin, D. Benardot, Å. B. Tornberg, S. Skouby, J. Faber, J. K.undgot-Borgen, and A. K. Melin. "Within-Day Energy Deficiency and Reproductive Function in Female Endurance Athletes." *Scandinavian Journal of Medicine & Science in Sports* 28, no. 3 (2018): 1139–46. https://pubmed.ncbi.nlm.nih.gov/29205517.

Fazal, Wahab, Atika Bibi, Ullah Farhad, Shahab Muhammad, and Behr Rüdiger. "Metabolic Impact on the Hypothalamic Kisspeptin-Kiss1r Signaling Pathway." *Frontiers in Endocrinology* 9 (March 2018). www .frontiersin.org/articles/10.3389/fendo.2018.00123/full.

Gregorio, L., J. Brindisi, A. Kleppinger, R. Sullivan, K. M. Mangano, J. D. Bihuniak, A. M. Kenny, J. E. Kerstetter, and K. L. Insogna. "Adequate Dietary Protein Is Associated with Better Physical Performance Among Post-Menopausal Women 60–90 Years." *Journal of Nutrition, Health & Aging* 18, no. 2 (2014): 155–160. www.ncbi .nlm.nih.gov/pmc/articles/PMC4433492.

Heikura, Ida A., Louise M. Burke, John A. Hawley, Megan L. Ross, Laura Garvican-Lewis, Avish P. Sharma, Alannah K. A. McKay, et al. "A Short-Term Ketogenic Diet Impairs Markers of Bone Health in Response to Exercise." *Frontiers in Endocrinology* 10 (January 2020). www.frontiersin.org/articles/10.3389/fendo.2019.00880 /full.

Heilbronn, Leonie K., Anthony E. Civitarese, Iwona Bogacka, Steven R. Smith, Matthew Hulver, Eric Ravussin. "Glucose Tolerance and Skeletal Muscle Gene Expression in Response to Alternate Day Fasting." *Obesity* 13, no. 3 (2005): 574–81. https://onlinelibrary.wiley.com/doi/full/10.1038/oby.2005.61.

Holcomb, Lola E., Caitlin C. O'Neill, Elizabeth A. DeWitt, and Stephen C. Kolwicz Jr. "The Effects of Fasting or Ketogenic Diet on Endurance Exercise Performance and Metabolism in Female Mice." *Metabolites* 11, no. 6 (2021): 397. www.mdpi.com/2218-1989/11/6/397.

Kassab, Salah E., Tarik Abdul-Ghaffar, Das S. Nagalla, Usha Sachdeva, and Usha Nayar. "Serum Leptin and Insulin Levels During Chronic Diurnal Fasting." *Asia Pacific Journal of Clinical Nutrition* 12, no. 4 (2003): 483–87. https://pubmed.ncbi.nlm.nih.gov/14672875.

Lagou, Vasiliki, Reedik Mägi, Jouke- Jan Hottenga, Harald Grallert, John R. B. Perry, Nabila Bouatia-Naji, Letizia Marullo, Denis Rybin, Rick Jansen, et al. "Sex-Dimorphic Genetic Effects and Novel Loci for Fasting Glucose and Insulin Variability." *Nature Communications* 12, 24 (2021). www.nature.com/articles/s41467-020 -19366-9.

Navarro, Victor M. "Metabolic Regulation of Kisspeptin: The Link Between Energy Balance and Reproduction." *Nature Reviews Endocrinology* 16 (2020): 407–20. www.nature.com/articles/s41574-020-0363-7.

P, Verma, and Dikansha Trikha. "Review on Role of Ketogenic Diet and Excessive Workout on Hormonal Imbalances in Women." *Journal of Obesity & Weight Loss Therapy* 8, no. 4 (2018). www.researchgate.net /publication/328283264_Review_on_Role_of_Ketogenic_ Diet_and_Excessive_Workout_on_Hormonal _Imbalances_in_Women.

Parr, Evelyn B., Leonie K. Heilbronn, John A. Hawley. "A Time to Eat and a Time to Exercise." *Exercise and Sport Sciences Reviews* 48, no. 1 (2020): 4–10. https://pubmed.ncbi.nlm.nih.gov/31688298.

Piotrowska, Katarzyna, Maciej Tarnowski, Katarzyna Zgutka, and Andrzej Pawlik. "Gender Differences in Response to Prolonged Every-Other-Day Feeding on the Proliferation and Apoptosis of Hepatocytes in Mice." *Nutrients* 8, no. 3 (2016): 176. https://doi.org/10.3390/nu8030176.

Santos, Heitor O., and Rodrigo C. O. Macedo. "Impact of Intermittent Fasting on the Lipid Profile: Assessment Associated with Diet and Weight Loss." *Clinical Nutrition ESPEN* 24 (January 2018): 14–21. https://doi.org/10 .1016/j.clnesp.2018.01.002.

Sjödin, Anna, Fredrik Hellström, EwaCarin Sehlstedt, Michael Svensson, and Jonas Burén. "Effects of a Ketogenic Diet on Muscle Fatigue in Healthy, Young, Normal-Weight Women: A Randomized Controlled Feeding Trial." *Nutrients* 12, no. 4 (2020): 955. www.mdpi.com/2072-6643/12/4/955.

Stannard, Stephen R., Alex J. Buckley, Johann A. Edge, Martin W. Thompson. "Adaptations to Skeletal Muscle with Endurance Exercise Training in the Acutely Fed Versus Overnight-Fasted State." *Journal of Science and Medicine in Sport* 13, no. 4 (2010). www.jsams.org/article/S1440-2440(10)00073-3/fulltext.

Tao, Zhipeng, Limin Shi, Jane Parke, Louise Zheng, Wei Gu, X. Charlie Dong, Dongmin Liu, Zongwei Wang, Aria F. Olumi, and Zhiyong Cheng. "Sirt1 Coordinates with ERα to Regulate Autophagy and Adiposity." *Cell Death Discovery* 5, no. 53 (2021). www.nature.com/articles/s41420-021-00438-8.

Wang, Lijun, Jiaqi Wang, Dragos Cretoiu, Guoping Li, and JunjieXiao. "Exercise-Mediated Regulation of Autophagy in the Cardiovascular System." *Journal of Sport and Health Science* 9, no. 3 (2020): 203–10. www .sciencedirect.com/science/article/pii/S2095254619301310?via%3Dihub.

Wasserfurth, Paulina, Jana Palmowski, Andreas Hahn, and Karsten Krüge. "Reasons for and Consequences of Low Energy Availability in Female and Male Athletes: Social Environment, Adaptations, and Prevention." *Sports Medicine – Open* 6, no. 44 (2020). https://sportsmedicine-open.springeropen.com/articles/10.1186/s40798 -020-00275-6.

10: FUELING FOR THE MENOPAUSE TRANSITION

Jackman, Sarah R., Oliver C. Witard, Andrew Philp, Gareth A. Wallis, Keith Baar, and Kevin D. Tipton. "Branched-Chain Amino Acid Ingestion Stimulates Muscle Myofibrillar Protein Synthesis following Resistance Exercise in Humans." *Frontiers in Physiology* 8 (June 2017). www.frontiersin.org/articles/10.3389/fphys.2017.00390/full.

Shanmugalingam, Thurkaa, Cecilia Bosco, Anne J. Ridley, and Mieke Van Hemelrijck. "Is There a Role for IGF-1 in the Development of Second Primary Cancers?" *Cancer Medicine* 5, no. 11 (2016): 3353–67. www.ncbi.nlm.nih .gov/pmc/articles/PMC5119990.

11: NAIL YOUR NUTRITION TIMING

Gorissen, Stefan H. M., Julie J. R. Crombag, Joan M. G. Senden, W. A. Huub Waterval, Jörgen Bierau, Lex B. Verdijk, and Luc J. C. van Loon. "Protein Content and Amino Acid Composition of Commercially Available Plant-Based Protein Isolates." *Amino Acids* 50, no. 12 (2018): 1685–95. www.ncbi.nlm.nih.gov/pmc/articles /PMC6245118.

Kealey J. Wohlgemuth, Kealey J., Luke R. Arieta, Gabrielle J. Brewer, Andrew L. Hoselton, Lacey M. Gould, and Abbie E. Smith-Ryan. "Sex Differences and Considerations for Female Specific Nutritional Strategies: A Narrative Review." *Journal of the International Society of Sports Nutrition* 18 (April 2021). https://jissn .biomedcentral.com/articles/10.1186/s12970-021-00422-8.

12: HOW TO HYDRATE

Aiko Wickham, Kate Aiko, Devin G. McCarthy, Lawrence L. Spriet, and Stephen S. Cheung. "Sex Differences in the Physiological Responses to Exercise-Induced Dehydration: Consequences and Mechanisms?" *Journal of Applied Physiology* 131, no. 2 (2021): 504–10. https://journals.physiology.org/doi/prev/20210701-aop/abs/10.1152 /japplphysiol.00266.2021.

Lertrit, Amornpan, Sasinee Srimachai, Sunee Saetung, Suwannee Chanprasertyothin, La-or Chailurkit, Chatvara Areevut, Pornalat Katekao, Boonsong Ongphiphadhanakul, and Chutintorn Sriphrapradang. "Effects of Sucralose on Insulin and Glucagon-Like Peptide-1 Secretion in Healthy Subjects: A Randomized, Double-Blind, Placebo-Controlled Trial." *Nutrition* 55–56 (April 2018): 125–30. https://pubmed.ncbi.nlm.nih.gov/30005329.

Stachenfeld, Nina S. "Hormonal Changes During Menopause and the Impact on Fluid Regulation." *Reproductive Sciences* 21, no. 5 (2014): 555–61. www.ncbi.nlm.nih.gov/pmc/articles/PMC3984489.

13: SLEEP WELL AND RECOVER RIGHT

Losso, Jack N., John W. Finley, Namrata Karki, Ann G. Liu, Weihong Pan, Alfredo Prudente, Russell Tipton, Ying Yu, and Frank L. Greenway. "Pilot Study of Tart Cherry Juice for the Treatment of Insomnia and Investigation of Mechanisms." *American Journal of Therapeutics* 25, no. 2 (2018): e194–3201. www.ncbi.nlm.nih.gov/pmc/articles/PMC5617749.

Muqeet Adnan, Mohammed, Muhammad Khan, Syed Hashmi, Muhammad Hamza, Sufyan AbdulMujeeb, and Syed Amer. "Black Cohosh and Liver Toxicity: Is There a Relationship?" *Case Reports in Gastrointestinal Medicine* 2014 (June 2014): 860614. www.ncbi.nlm.nih.gov/pmc/articles/PMC4100270.

Newton, Katherine M., Susan D. Reed, Katherine A. Guthrie, Karen J. Sherman, Cathryn Booth-LaForce, Bette Caan, and Barbara Sternfeld. "Efficacy of Yoga for Vasomotor Symptoms: A Randomized Controlled Trial." *Menopause* 21, no. 4 (2014): 339–46. www.ncbi.nlm.nih.gov/pmc/articles/PMC3871975.

Reed, Susan D., Katherine A. Guthrie, Katherine M. Newton, Garnet L. Anderson, Cathryn Booth-LaForce, Bette Caan, and Janet S. Carpenter. "Menopausal Quality of Life: RCT of Yoga, Exercise, and Omega-3 Supplements." *Research Reproductive Endocrinology and Infertility* 210, no. 3 (2014): 244.e1–244.e11. www.ajog.org/article/S0002-9378(13)02015-2/fulltext.

Shinjyo, Noriko, Guy Waddell, and Julia Green. "Valerian Root in Treating Sleep Problems and Associated Disorders—A Systematic Review and Meta-Analysis." *Journal of Evidence-Based Integrative Medicine* 25 (October 2020). www.ncbi.nlm.nih.gov/pmc/articles/PMC7585905.

Van Cauter, Eve, Kristen Knutson, Rachel Leproult, and Karine Spiegel. "The Impact of Sleep Deprivation on Hormones and Metabolism." *Medscape Neurology* 7, no. 1 (2005). www.medscape.org/viewarticle/502825.

Wang, Ximei; Shuyi Wang, Huan Wu, Mingfei Jiang, Hui Xue, Yangqi Zhu, Chenxu Wang, Xiaojuan Zha, Yufeng Wen. "Human Growth Hormone Level Decreased in Women Aged <60 Years but Increased in Men Aged >50 Years." *Medicine* 99, no. 2 (2020): e18440. www.ncbi.nlm.nih.gov/pmc/articles/PMC6959966.

14: STABILITY, MOBILITY, AND CORE STRENGTH: KEEP YOUR FOUNDATION STRONG

Chlebowski, Rowan T., Dominic J. Cirillo, Charles B. Eaton, Marcia L. Stefanick, Mary Pettinger, Laura D. Carbone, Karen C. Johnson, Michael S. Simon, Nancy F. Woods, and Jean Wactawski-Wende. "Estrogen Alone and Joint Symptoms in the Women's Health Initiative Randomized Trial." *Menopause* 25, no. 11 (2018): 1313–20. https://pubmed.ncbi.nlm.nih.gov/30358728.

Jin, X., B. H. Wang, X. Wang, B. Antony, Z. Zhu, W. Han, F. Cicuttini, et al. "Associations Between Endogenous Sex Hormones and MRI Structural Changes in Patients with Symptomatic Knee Osteoarthritis." *Osteoarthritis and Cartilage* 25, no. 7 (2017): 1100–1106. www.sciencedirect.com/science/article/pii/S1063458417300468.

15: MOTIVATION AND THE MENTAL GAME: MIND YOUR MATTERS

Jacobs, Emily G., Blair K. Weiss, Nikos Makris, Sue Whitfield-Gabrieli, Stephen L. Buka, Anne Klibanski, and Jill M. Goldstein. "Impact of Sex and Menopausal Status on Episodic Memory Circuitry in Early Midlife." *Journal of Neuroscience* 36, no. 39 (2016): 10163–73. www.jneurosci.org/content/36/39/10163.long.

Konishi, Kyoko, Sara Cherkerzian, SarahAroner, Emily G. Jacobs, Dorene M.Rentz, Anne Remington, Harlyn Aizley, Mady Hornig, Anne Klibanski, Jill M. Goldstein. "Impact of BDNF and Sex on Maintaining Intact Memory Function in Early Midlife." *Neurobiology of Aging* 88 (April 2020): 137–49. www.sciencedirect.com/science/article/abs/pii/S0197458019304427.

Kujach, Sylwester, Robert Antoni Olek, Kyeongho Byun, Kazuya Suwabe, Emilia J. Sitek, Ewa Ziemann, Radosław Laskowski, and Hideaki Soya. "Acute Sprint Interval Exercise Increases Both Cognitive Functions and Peripheral Neurotrophic Factors in Humans: The Possible Involvement of Lactate." *Frontiers in Neuroscience* 13 (January 2020). www.ncbi.nlm.nih.gov/pmc/articles/PMC6989590.

Lejri, Imane, Amandine Grimm, and Anne Eckert. "Mitochondria, Estrogen and Female Brain Aging." *Frontiers in Aging Neuroscience* 10 (April 2018). www.frontiersin.org/articles/10.3389/fnagi.2018.00124/full.

16: KEEP YOUR SKELETON STRONG

Alejandro Gómez-Bruton, Alejandro Gónzalez-Agüero, Alba Gómez-Cabello, José A. Casajús, and Germán Vicente-Rodríguez. "Is Bone Tissue Really Affected by Swimming? A Systematic Review." *PLoS One* 8, no. 8 (2013): e70119. www.ncbi.nlm.nih.gov/pmc/articles/PMC3737199.

Capozzi, Anna, Giovanni Scambia, and Stefano Lello. "Calcium, Vitamin D, Vitamin K2, and Magnesium Supplementation and Skeletal Health." *Maturitas* 140 (October 2020): 55–63. https://pubmed.ncbi.nlm.nih.gov /32972636.

Follis, Shawna L., Jennifer Bea, Yann Klimentidis, Chengcheng Hu, C. J. Crandall, David O. Garcia, Aladdin H. Shadyab, Rami Nassir, and Zhao Chen. "Psychosocial Stress and Bone Loss Among Postmenopausal Women: Results from the Women's Health Initiative." *Journal of Epidemiology and Community Health* 73, no. 9 (2019):888–92. https://jech.bmj.com/content/73/9/888.

Hind, Karen. Hind, Karen. "Recovery of Bone Mineral Density and Fertility in a Former Amenorrheic Athlete." *Journal of Sports Science & Medicine* 7, no. 3 (2018): 415–18. www.ncbi.nlm.nih.gov/pmc/articles/PMC3761891.

Ross, A. Catharine, JoAnn E. Manson, Steven A. Abrams, John F. Aloia, Patsy M. Brannon, Steven K. Clinton, Ramon A. Durazo-Arvizu, et al. "The 2011 Report on Dietary Reference Intakes for Calcium and Vitamin D from the Institute of Medicine: What Clinicians Need to Know." *Journal of Clinical Endocrinology and Metabolism* 96, no. 1 (2011): 53–58. www.ncbi.nlm.nih.gov/pmc/articles/PMC3046611.

Watson, Steven L., Benjamin K. Weeks, Lisa J. Weis, Amy T. Harding, Sean A. Horan, Belinda R. Beck. "High-Intensity Resistance and Impact Training Improves Bone Mineral Density and Physical Function in Postmenopausal Women with Osteopenia and Osteoporosis: The LIFTMOR Randomized Controlled Trial." *Journal of Bone and Mineral Research* 33, no. 2 (2018): 211–20. https://asbmr.onlinelibrary.wiley.com/doi/full/10 .1002/jbmr.3284.

17: STRATEGIES FOR EXERCISING THROUGH THE TRANSITION

"ACOG Committee Opinion No. 659: The Use of Vaginal Estrogen in Women with a History of Estrogen-Dependent Breast Cancer." *Obstetrics and Gynecology* 127, no. 3 (2016): e93–e96. https://pubmed.ncbi.nlm.nih .gov/26901334.

Fedewa, Michael V., Steven O. Spencer, Tyler D. Williams, Zachery E. Becker, and Collin A. Fuqua. "Effect of Branched-Chain Amino Acid Supplementation on Muscle Soreness Following Exercise: A Meta-Analysis." *International Journal for Vitamin and Nutrition Research* 89, no. 5–6 (2019): 348–56. https://pubmed.ncbi.nlm .nih.gov/30938579.

Kato, Hiroyuki, Hiromi Suzuki, Masako Mimura, Yoshiko Inoue, Mayu Sugita, Katsuya Suzuki, and Hisamine Kobayashi. "Leucine-Enriched Essential Amino Acids Attenuate Muscle Soreness and Improve Muscle Protein Synthesis After Eccentric Contractions in Rats." *Amino Acids* 47, no. 6 (2015): 1193–1201. www.ncbi.nlm.nih.gov /pmc/articles/PMC4429140.

Nicol, Lesley M., David S. Rowlands, Ruth Fazakerly, and John Kellett. "Curcumin Supplementation Likely Attenuates Delayed Onset Muscle Soreness (DOMS)." *European Journal of Applied Physiology* 115, no. 8 (2015): 1769–77. https://pubmed.ncbi.nlm.nih.gov/25795285.

Woods, Rosanne, Rebecca Hess, Carol Biddington, and Marc Federico. "Association of Lean Body Mass to Menopausal Symptoms: The Study of Women's Health Across the Nation." *Women's Midlife Health* 6, no. 10 (2020). https://womensmidlifehealthjournal.biomedcentral.com/articles/10.1186/s40695-020-00058-9.

18: SUPPLEMENTS: WHAT YOU NEED AND WHAT YOU DON'T

Abbasi, Behnood, Masud Kimiagar, Khosro Sadeghniiat, Minoo M. Shirazi, Mehdi Hedayati, and Bahram Rashidkhani. "The Effect of Magnesium Supplementation on Primary Insomnia in Elderly: A Double-Blind Placebo-Controlled Clinical Trial." *Journal of Research in Medical Sciences* 17, no. 2 (2012): 1161–69. www.ncbi .nlm.nih.gov/pmc/articles/PMC3703169.

Alfaro-Magallanes, Víctor M., Pedro J. Benito, Beatriz Rael, Laura Barba-Moreno, Nuria Romero-Parra, Rocío Cupeiro, Dorine W. Swinkels, Coby M. Laarakkers, Ana B. Peinado, and on behalf of the IronFEMME Study

Group. "Menopause Delays the Typical Recovery of Pre-Exercise Hepcidin Levels after High-Intensity Interval Running Exercise in Endurance-Trained Women." *Nutrients* 12, no. 12 (2020): 3866. www.ncbi.nlm.nih.gov /pmc/articles/PMC7766833.

Bacchetta, Justine, Joshua J. Zaritsky, Jessica L. Sea, Rene F. Chun, Thomas S. Lisse, Kathryn Zavala, Anjali Nayak, et al. "Suppression of Iron-Regulatory Hepcidin by Vitamin D." *Journal of American Society of Nephrology* 25, no. 3 (2014): 564–72. https://jasn.asnjournals.org/content/25/3/564#:~:text=VitaminDsuppressesexpressionof ,inhumanmonocytesandhepatocytes.

Burt, Lauren A., Emma O. Billington, Marianne S. Rose, Duncan A. Raymond, David A. Hanley, and Steven K. Boyd. "Effect of High-Dose Vitamin D Supplementation on Volumetric Bone Density and Bone Strength: A Randomized Clinical Trial." *JAMA* 322, no. 8 (2019): 736–45. https://jamanetwork.com/journals/jama /fullarticle/2748796.

Cameron, Donnie, Ailsa A. Welch, Fatemeh Adelnia, Christopher M. Bergeron, David A. Reiter, Ligia J. Dominguez, Nicholas A. Brennan, Kenneth W. Fishbein, Richard G. Spencer, and Luigi Ferrucci. "Age and Muscle Function Are More Closely Associated with Intracellular Magnesium, As Assessed by 31P Magnetic Resonance Spectroscopy, Than with Serum Magnesium." *Frontiers in Physiology* 10 (November 2019): 1454. www.frontiersin.org/articles/10.3389/fphys.2019.01454/full.

Dahlquist, Dylan T., Brad P. Dieter, and Michael S. Koeh. "Plausible Ergogenic Effects of Vitamin D on Athletic Performance and Recovery." *Journal of the International Society of Sports Nutrition* 12 (August 2015). https://jissn .biomedcentral.com/articles/10.1186/s12970-015-0093-8.

Eckerson, Joan M. "Creatine as an Ergogenic Aid for Female Athletes." *Strength and Conditioning Journal* 38, no. 2 (2016): 14–23. https://journals.lww.com/nsca-scj/Fulltext/2016/04000/Creatine_as_an_Ergogenic_Aid_for _Female_Athletes.4.aspx.

Ellery, Stacey J., David W. Walker, and Hayley Dickinson. "Creatine for Women: a Review of the Relationship Between Creatine and the Reproductive Cycle and Female-Specific Benefits of Creatine Therapy." *Amino Acids* 48 (February 2016): 1807–17. https://link.springer.com/article/10.1007%2Fs00726-016-2199-y.

Glenn, J. M., M. Gray, R. Stewart, N. E. Moyen, S. A. Kavouras, R. DiBrezzo, R. Turner, R., and J. Baum. "Incremental Effects of 28 Days of Beta-Alanine Supplementation on High-Intensity Cycling Performance and Blood Lactate in Masters Female Cyclists." *Amino Acids* 47, no. 12 (2015): 2593–2600. https://pubmed.ncbi.nlm .nih.gov/26255281.

Glenn, Jordan M., Michelle Gray, Bruno Gualano, and Hamilton Roschel. "The Ergogenic Effects of Supplemental Nutritional Aids on Anaerobic Performance in Female Athletes." *Strength and Conditioning Journal* 38, no. 2 (2016): 105–120. https://journals.lww.com/nsca-scj/Fulltext/2016/04000/The_Ergogenic_Effects_of_ Supplemental_Nutritional.15.aspx.

Glenn, Jordan M., Michelle Gray, Rodger W. Stewart Jr., Nicole E. Moyen, Stavros A. Kavouras, Ro DiBrezzo, Ronna Turner, Jamie I Baum, and Matthew S. Stone. "Effects of 28-Day Beta-Alanine Supplementation on Isokinetic Exercise Performance and Body Composition in Female Masters Athletes." *Journal of Strength and Conditioning Research* 30, no. 1 (2016): 200–207. https://pubmed.ncbi.nlm.nih.gov/26110349.

Goodman, Gary E., Mark D. Thornquist, John Balmes, Mark R. Cullen, Frank L. Meyskens Jr., Gilbert S. Omenn, Barbara Valanis, James H. Williams Jr. "The Beta-Carotene and Retinol Efficacy Trial: Incidence of Lung Cancer and Cardiovascular Disease Mortality During 6-Year Follow-up After Stopping β-Carotene and Retinol Supplements." *Journal of the National Cancer Institute* 96, no. 23 (2004): 1743–50. https://academic.oup.com /jnci/article/96/23/1743/2521077.

Guest, Nanci S., Trisha A. VanDusseldorp, Michael T. Nelson, Jozo Grgic, Brad J. Schoenfeld, Nathaniel D. M. Jenkins, Shawn M. Arent, et al. "International Society of Sports Nutrition Position Stand: Caffeine and Exercise Performance." *Journal of the International Society of Sports Nutrition* 18 (January 2021). https://jissn .biomedcentral.com/articles/10.1186/s12970-020-00383-4.

Jian, Jinlong, Edward Pelle, and Xi Huang. "Iron and Menopause: Does Increased Iron Affect the Health of Postmenopausal Women?" *Antioxidants & Redox Signaling* 11, no. 12 (2009): 2939–43. www.ncbi.nlm.nih.gov /pmc/articles/PMC2821138.

Kasprowicz, Katarzyna, Wojciech Ratkowski, Wojciech Wołyniec, Mariusz Kaczmarczyk, Konrad Witek, Piotr Żmijewski, Marcin Renke, et al. "The Effect of Vitamin D3 Supplementation on Hepcidin, Iron, and IL-6 Responses After a 100 km Ultra-Marathon." *International Journal of Environmental Research and Public Health* 17, no. 8: 2962. www.ncbi.nlm.nih.gov/pmc/articles/PMC7215841.

Lis, Dana M., and Keith Baar. "Effects of Different Vitamin C–Enriched Collagen Derivatives on Collagen Synthesis." *International Journal of Sport Nutrition and Exercise Metabolism* 29, no. 5 (2019): 526–31. https://journals.humankinetics.com/view/journals/ijsnem/29/5/article-p526.xml?content=abstract.

Lyoo, Kyoon, Sujung Yoon, Tae-Suk Kim, Jaeuk Hwang, Jieun E. Kim, Wangyoun Won, Sujin Bae, and Perry F. Renshaw. "A Randomized, Double-Blind Placebo-Controlled Trial of Oral Creatine Monohydrate Augmentation for Enhanced Response to a Selective Serotonin Reuptake Inhibitor in Women with Major Depressive Disorder." *American Journal of Psychiatry* 169, no. 9 (2012): 937–45. https://ajp.psychiatryonline.org/doi/full/10.1176/appi.ajp.2012.12010009.

Marks, Robin, Peter A. Foley, Damien Jolley, Kenneth R. Knight, Josephine Harrison, and Sandra C. Thompson. "The Effect of Regular Sunscreen Use on Vitamin D Levels in an Australian Population: Results of a Randomized Controlled Trial." *Archives of Dermatology* 131, no. 4 (1995): 415–21. https://jamanetwork.com/journals/jamadermatology/article-abstract/556563.

Pasricha, Sant-Rayn, Michael Low, Jane Thompson, Ann Farrell, and Luz-Maria De-Regil. "Iron Supplementation Benefits Physical Performance in Women of Reproductive Age: A Systematic Review and Meta-Analysis." *Journal of Nutrition* 144, no. 6 (2014): 906–14. https://academic.oup.com/jn/article/144/6/906/4616008.

Robbins, John A., Aaron Aragaki, Carolyn J. Crandall, Joann E. Manson, Laura Carbone, Rebecca Jackson, Cora E. Lewis, et al. "Women's Health Initiative Clinical Trials: Interaction of Calcium Plus Vitamin D and Hormone Therapy." *Menopause* 21, no. 2 (2014): 116–23. www.ncbi.nlm.nih.gov/pmc/articles/PMC3830603.

Rosanoff, Andrea, Connie M. Weaver, and Robert K. Rude. "Suboptimal Magnesium Status in the United States: Are the Health Consequences Underestimated?" *Nutrition Reviews* 70, no. 3 (2012): 153–64. https://pubmed.ncbi.nlm.nih.gov/22364157.

Smith-Ryan, Abbie E., Hannah E. Cabre, Joan M. Eckerson, and Darren G. Candow. "Creatine Supplementation in Women's Health: A Lifespan Perspective." *Nutrients* 13, no. 3 (2021): 877. www.mdpi.com/2072-6643/13/3/877.

Stoffel, Nicole U., Christophe Zeder, Gary M. Brittenham, Diego Moretti, and Michael B. Zimmermann. "Iron Absorption from Supplements Is Greater with Alternate Day Than with Consecutive Day Dosing in Iron-Deficient Anemic Women." *Haematologica* 105, no. 5 (2020): 1232–39. www.ncbi.nlm.nih.gov/pmc/articles/PMC7193469/#:~:text=Inirondepletedwomenwithout,isgivenonalternatedays.

Trexler, Eric T., Abbie E. Smith-Ryan, Jeffrey R. Stout, Jay R. Hoffman, Colin D. Wilborn, Craig Sale, Richard B. Kreider, et al. "International Society of Sports Nutrition Position Stand: Beta-Alanine." *Journal of the International Society of Sports Nutrition* 12 (July 2021). www.ncbi.nlm.nih.gov/pmc/articles/PMC4501114.

Welch, Ailsa a., Eirini Kelaiditi, Amy Jennings, Claire J. Steves, Tim D. Spector, and Alexander Macgregor. "Dietary Magnesium Is Positively Associated with Skeletal Muscle Power and Indices of Muscle Mass and May Attenuate the Association Between Circulating C-Reactive Protein and Muscle Mass in Women." *Journal of Bone and Mineral Research* 31, no 2 (2016): 317–25. https://pubmed.ncbi.nlm.nih.gov/26288012.

Yerushalmi, Rinat, Sharon Bargil, Yaara Ber, Rachel Ozlavo, Tuval Sivan, Yael Rapson, Adi Pomerantz, et al. "3,3-Diindolylmethane (DIM): A Nutritional Intervention and Its Impact on Breast Density in Healthy BRCA Carriers; a Prospective Clinical Trial." *Carcinogenesis* 41, no. 10 (2020): 1395–1401. https://academic.oup.com/carcin/article/41/10/1395/5847633.

19: PULLING IT ALL TOGETHER

Flegal, Katherine M., Brian K. Kit, Heather Orpana, and Barry I. Garubard. "Association of All-Cause Mortality with Overweight and Obesity Using Standard Body Mass Index Categories: A Systematic Review and Meta-Analysis." *JAMA* 309, no. 1 (2013): 71–82. https://pubmed.ncbi.nlm.nih.gov/23280227.

Ramos-Jiménez, Arnulfo, Rebeca Chávez-Herrera, Aida S. Castro-Sosa, Lilia C. Pérez-Hernández, Rosa P. Hernández Torres, and David Olivas-Dávila. "Body Shape, Image, and Composition as Predictors of Athlete's Performance." Chapter 2 in *Fitness Medicine,* edited by Hasan Sozen. Rijeka, Croatia: IntechOpen, 2016. www .intechopen.com/books/fitness-medicine/body-shape-image-and-composition-as-predictors-of-athlete-s -performance.

Ryan-Stewart, Helen, James Faulkner, and Simon Jobson. "the Influence of Somatotype on Anaerobic Performance." *PLoS One* 13, no. 5 (2018). www.ncbi.nlm.nih.gov/pmc/articles/PMC5963773.

INDEX

nonprescription hormones, 60–61

norepinephrine, 61–62

nutrition, 140–157, 158–173. *See also* timing of eating
    background, 158–159
    for bone health, 250–251
    calorie recommendations, 159–160
    cruciferous vegetables, 164–165
    energy availability and, 142–147
    hydration recommendations, 172–173, 287
    injury comebacks and, 219
    intermittent fasting, 152, 153–154
    keto diet, 152, 154–156
    leucine, 171–172
    low energy availability, 140–142, 144, 145–147,
        176–177
    macronutrient recommendations, 160–164,
        166–170
    Next Level Makeover, 65, 147–151
    planning, 285–290
    plant-based eating, 156–157, 166–168,
        177–178
    processed foods, 130, 139, 178
    super-smoothies, 168
    sweeteners, 139, 162, 196–197
    training gains through, 151–152
    vitamins and minerals, 165–166, 250–251, 265–271.
        See also supplements

Obama, Michelle, 14

omega-3 fatty acids, 219–220, 251, 256, 262

oral contraceptives, 59–60

osteoporosis, 248, 251–253. *See also* bone strength and
    density

Oura Ring, 39, 201–202

pelvic floor exercises, 97–98

performance-enhancing compounds, 271–276

perimenopause, 16–18

"period underwear," 257

periods, 45–46, 59–60, 141, 246, 256–257

Peruvian ginseng (maca root), 73–74

picoAMH Elisa diagnostic test, 19, 20

plan of action
    1. track the changes, 277–278
    2. take symptom inventory, 278–280
    3. track body composition, 281–284
    4. schedule your training, 284–285
    5. planning your nutrition, 285–290

plant-based eating, 156–157, 166–168,
    177–178

plyometrics, 113–123
    aqua jumping, 123
    background, 113–114
    benefits of, 36, 114–116
    how to, 116–123
    stability and posture for, 223

PMS symptoms, 256–257

posture, 108–109, 223, 249

prebiotics, 129–130, 136–137, 165

Premarin, 60

probiotics, 129, 130

processed foods, 130, 139, 178

progesterone
    function of, 30, 32–33, 36–42, 43–44
    medical uses, 57–58
    menopause testing and, 19–20
    sleep and, 202–203
    stability and, 221–222
    symptoms related to levels of,
        258–259

progestin pills, 46, 59–60, 256

protein
    -carbohydrate combinations, 169–170
    energy availability and, 144
    following training sessions, 166–167
    for injury comebacks, 219, 220
    intake recommendations, 161–162, 166–167, 171–172,
        177–178, 287–289
    plant-based, 166–168, 177–178

protein powders, 166

race and ethnicity differences, 12–13, 22–24,
    253

reactive oxygen species (ROS), 32

recovery techniques and tracking, 201–202, 210–214,
    262–263

relative energy deficiency in sport (RED-S), 141–142, 144,
    145–147, 246

Rhodiola rosea, 70–71

Rowan, Lynda, 237

RPE (rating of perceived exertion) scale, 86

Rusch, Rebecca, 4, 78

salt, 189–190, 191–192

satiety, 33–34

schisandra (Magnolia berry), 71, 72–73

Veillonella, 131
vitamin and mineral recommendations, 165–166, 250–
      251, 265–271. *See also* supplements; *specific
      vitamins and minerals*
vitamin C, 268
vitamin D, 250, 251, 265–267, 268
vitamin K2, 250–251

weight gain, 43–45, 283. *See also* body
      composition

whey, 169, 177, 178, 219
Whoop Strap, 39, 67, 201–202
Wie, Michelle, 198
Wilson, Robert, 10
Winfrey, Oprah, 14
Winter, W. Christopher, 199, 200

Yeager, Selene, vii–ix, 136–137, 196, 241,
      242–243
yoga, 48, 161, 208

Also by STACY SIMS, PhD

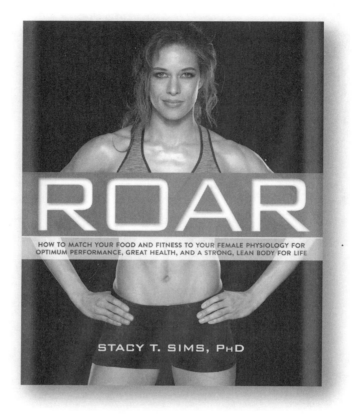

"Dr. Sims has taken her years of experience as an endurance
athlete and scientist to create the ultimate guide to nutrition and
performance for female athletes. No matter what your sport of choice is,
Roar is a book that no athlete should be without."

—SHALUINN FULLOVE, two-time U.S. Olympic Marathon Trials qualifier